Ranger Medic Handbook

U.S. Department of Defense

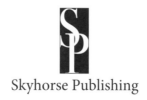

Skyhorse Publishing

Visit our website at www.skyhorsepublishing.com.

10 9 8

Library of Congress Cataloging-in-Publication Data is available on file.

Cover design by Rain Saukas

ISBN: 978-1-63450-332-7
Ebook ISBN: 978-1-63450-959-6
Printed in China

Ranger Medic Handbook

FOREWORD

Historically in warfare, the majority of all combat deaths have occurred prior to a casualty ever receiving advanced trauma management. The execution of the Ranger mission profile in the Global War on Terrorism and our legacy tasks undoubtedly will increase the number of lethal wounds.

Ranger leaders can significantly reduce the number of Rangers who die of wounds sustained in combat by simply targeting optimal medical capability in close proximity to the point of wounding. Survivability of the traumatized Ranger who sustains a wound in combat is in the hands of the first responding Ranger who puts a pressure dressing or tourniquet and controls the bleeding of his fallen comrade. Directing casualty response management and evacuation is a Ranger leader task; ensuring technical medical competence is a Ranger Medic task.

A solid foundation has been built for Ranger leaders and medics to be successful in managing casualties in a combat environment. An integrated team response from non-medical personnel and medical providers must be in place to care for the wounded Ranger. The Ranger First Responder, Squad EMT, Ranger Medic Advanced Tactical Practitioner, and Ranger leaders, in essence all Rangers must unite to provide medical care collectively, as a team, without sacrificing the flow and violence of the battle at hand.

An integrated team approach to casualty response and care will directly translate to the reduction of the died of wounds rate of combat casualties and minimize the turbulence associated with these events in times of crisis. The true success of the Ranger Medical Team will be defined by its ability to complete the mission and greatly reduce preventable combat death. Rangers value honor and reputation more than their lives, and as such will attempt to lay down their own lives in defense of their comrades. The Ranger Medic will do no less.

I will never leave a fallen comrade...

Harold R. Montgomery
MSG, USA
Regimental Senior Medic
1997-Present

RHHC Senior Medic
1995-1997
1/75 Plt, Co, BAS NCOIC
1990-1995

Russ S. Kotwal, MD
LTC, MC
Regimental Surgeon
2005-Present

3/75 Battalion Surgeon
1999-2003

Table of Contents

Subject	Page

Subject	Page

SECTION ONE

GENERAL OVERVIEW

MISSION STATEMENT

The mission of the 75th Ranger Regiment Trauma Management Team (Tactical) is to provide medical care and training in accordance with the tenets of Tactical Combat Casualty Care, Tactical Medical Emergency Protocols, and Pre-Hospital Trauma Life Support; in order to provide optimal health care to a Joint Special Operations Task Force conducting missions in support of U.S. policies and objectives.

RANGER MEDIC CHARTER

"SOCM ATP"
(Special Operations Combat Medic Advanced Tactical Practitioner)

Shoot and engage targets to defend casualties and self.

Operate relatively independently with highly-dispersed highly-mobile combat formations in an austere environment.

Communicate via secure and non-secure means.

Move tactically through unsecured areas.

Absolute master of the basics through pre-hospital trauma life support and tactical combat casualty care.

Timely, consistent, and competent provider of advanced trauma management within scope of practice.

Practitioner who assists licensed medical providers with medical emergencies and routine care encountered while in garrison, training, and during deployments.

REVIEW COMMITTEES

2001
MAJ Kotwal (3/75 Battalion Surgeon)
MAJ Meyer (3/75 Battalion PT)
CPT Detro (3/75 Battalion PA)
SFC Miller (3/75 Battalion Senior Medic)
SFC Montgomery (Regimental Senior Medic)
SSG Flores (3/75 Company Senior Medic)
SSG Gentry (3/75 Company Senior Medic)
SSG Muralles (3/75 Company Senior Medic)
SSG Odom (3/75 Company Senior Medic)
SSG Rothwell (3/75 Company Senior Medic)

2003
MAJ Wenzel (Regimental Surgeon)
MAJ Cain (1/75 Battalion Surgeon)
MAJ Kotwal (3/75 Battalion Surgeon)
MAJ Sassano (Regt Med Ops Officer)
SFC Montgomery (Regimental Senior Medic)
SFC Miller (Regt Med Plans & Trng NCO)
SFC Swain (2/75 Battalion Senior Medic)
SFC Flores (3/75 Battalion Senior Medic)
SSG Odom (3/75 Senior Medic)
SSG Williamson (2/75 Company Sr Medic)

2004
MAJ Wenzel (Regimental Surgeon)
CPT Pairmore (1/75 Battalion PA)
CPT Nieman (2/75 Battalion PA)
CPT Kelsey (Regt Med Ops Officer)
MSG Montgomery (Regt Senior Medic)
SFC Crays (2/75 Battalion Senior Medic)
SFC Flores (3/75 Battalion Senior Medic)
SSG Odom (3/75 Battalion Senior Medic)
SSG Williamson (Regt Med Training NCO)
SSG Medaris (1/75 Company Senior Medic)
SSG Garcia (2/75 Company Senior Medic)
SSG Severtson (2/75 Company Sr Medic)

2005
LTC Kotwal (Regimental Surgeon)
MAJ Matthews (1/75 Battalion Surgeon)
MAJ McCarver (2/75 Battalion Surgeon)
CPT Sterling (Regimental PA)
CPT Detro (3/75 Battalion PA)
CPT Reedy (1/75 Battalion PA)
CPT Slevin (2/75 Battalion PA)
CPT Grenier (2/75 Battalion PT)
CPT Soliz (3/160 Battalion PA)
MSG Montgomery (Regimental Senior Medic)
SFC Crays (2/75 Battalion Senior Medic)
SFC Warren (1/75 Battalion Senior Medic)
SSG Williamson (Regt Med Plans & Tng NCO)
SSG Gillaspie (2/75 Company Senior Medic)
SGT Kindig (2/75 Company Senior Medic)
SGT Robbins (3/75 Company Senior Medic)
SGT Slavens (3/75 Company Senior Medic)
SGT Morissette (3/75 Platoon Medic)
SPC Kacoroski (2/75 Platoon Medic)
SPC Ball (2/75 Platoon Medic)
SPC Lewis (3/75 Platoon Medic)
SPC Guadagnino (3/75 Platoon Medic)
SPC Drapeau (3/75 Platoon Medic)

2006
LTC Kotwal (Regimental Surgeon)
CPT Redman (1/75 Battalion Surgeon)
CPT Cunningham (2/75 Battalion Surgeon)
CPT Miles (3/75 Battalion Surgeon)
CPT Sterling (Regimental PA)
CPT Detro (Regimental PA)
CPT Fox (3/75 Battalion PA)
CPT Speer (Regt Med Ops Officer)
CPT Pollman (3/75 Battalion PT)
MSG Montgomery (Regimental Senior Medic)
SFC Odom (Regimental Medical Training NCO)
SSG Veliz (ROC Senior Medic)
SSG Garcia (2/75 Battalion Senior Medic)
SSG Williamson (3/75 Battalion Senior Medic)
SSG Gillaspie (2/75 Company Senior Medic)
SSG Bernas (2/75 Company Senior Medic)
SSG Chavaree (3/75 Company Senior Medic)
SSG Henigsmith (3/75 Company Senior Medic)
SGT Maitha (3/75 Company Senior Medic)

EDITORIAL CONSULTANTS

Executive Standing Members:
CAPT (Ret) Frank Butler, MD
CW4 (Ret) William Donovan, PA-C
COL John Holcomb, MD
LTC Russ Kotwal, MD, MPH
SFC (Ret) Robert Miller, NREMT
MSG Harold Montgomery, NREMT
Jeffrey Salomone, MD

Consulting & Contributing Members:
LTC Bret Ackermann, DO
MSG Perry Black, NREMT
CPT (Ret) Gregory Bromund, PA-C
LTC Brian Burlingame, MD
MAJ Jeffrey Cain, MD
CPT John Detro, PA-C
MAJ Arthur Finch, PhD
J.F. Rick Hammesfahr, MD
MAJ Shawn Kane, MD
MSG(Ret) Cory Lamoreaux, NREMT
LTC Robert Lutz, MD
MAJ Clinton Murray, MD
CPT (Ret) David Nieman, PA-C
LTC Kevin O'Connor, DO
CPT James Pairmore, PA-C
MAJ John Rayfield, MD
CPT Raymond Sterling, PA-C

Representative Organizations:
Committee on Tactical Combat Casualty Care
Defense and Veterans Brain Injury Center
Emory University Department of Surgery, Atlanta, GA
Grady Memorial Hospital, Atlanta, GA
Joint Special Operations Medical Training Center
PHTLS Committee of the NAEMT
US Army Institute of Surgical Research
US Special Operations Command State Department of EMS and Public Health

2007 Edition Chief Editors:
LTC Russ Kotwal, MD, MPH
MSG Harold Montgomery, NREMT, SOF-ATP

KEY REFERENCES

Texts:

1. **Advanced Trauma Life Support for Doctors**. 7th Edition, American College of Surgeons, Mosby, 2004.
2. **Basic and Advanced Prehospital Trauma Life Support: Military Edition**. Revised 5th Edition, National Association of Emergency Medical Technicians, Mosby, 2004.
3. **Emergency Medicine: A Comprehensive Study Guide**. 6th Edition, American College of Emergency Physicians, McGraw-Hill, 2004.
4. **Emergency War Surgery**. 3rd US Revision, Borden Institute, 2004.
5. **Griffith's Five-Minute Clinical Consult**. Lippincott, 2006.
6. **Guidelines for Field Management of Combat-Related Head Trauma**. Brain Trauma Foundation, 2005.
7. **Prentice Hall Nurse's Drug Guide**. Wilson, Shannon, and Stang, 2007.
8. **Tactical Medical Emergency Protocols for Special Operations Advanced Tactical Practitioners (ATPs)**. US Special Operations Command, 2006.
9. **Tarascon Adult Emergency Pocketbook**. 3rd Edition, Tarascon, 2005.
10. **Tarascon Pocket Pharmacopoeia**. Tarascon, 2006.
11. **The Sanford Guide to Antimicrobial Therapy**. 35th Edition, Antimicrobial Therapy, 2005.
12. **Wilderness Medicine**. 4th Edition, Mosby, 2001.

Articles:

1. Bellamy RF. **The causes of death in conventional land warfare: implications for combat casualty care research**. *Military Medicine*, 149:55, 1984.
2. Butler FK, Hagmann J, Butler EG. **Tactical Combat Casualty Care in Special Operations**. *Military Medicine*, 161(3 Suppl):1-15, 1996.
3. Butler FK Jr, Hagmann JH, Richards DT. **Tactical management of urban warfare casualties in special operations**. *Military Medicine*, 165(4 Suppl):1-48, 2000.
4. Holcomb JB. **Fluid resuscitation in modern Combat Casualty Care: lessons learned from Somalia**. *Journal of Trauma*, 54(5):46, 2003.
5. Kotwal RS, O'Connor KC, Johnson TR, Mosely DS, Meyer DE, Holcomb JB. **A novel pain management strategy for Combat Casualty Care**. *Annals of Emergency Medicine*, 44(2):121-7, 2004.
6. Lind GH, Marcus MA, Mears SL, et al. **Oral transmucosal fentanyl citrate for analgesia and sedation in the emergency department**. *Annals of Emergency Medicine*, 20(10):1117-20, 1991.
7. Murray CK, Hospenthal DR, Holcomb JB. **Antibiotic use and selection at the point of injury in Tactical Combat Casualty Care for casualties with penetrating abdominal injury, shock, or inability to tolerate oral agents**. *Journal of Special Operations Medicine*, 3(5):56-61, 2005.
8. O'Connor KC, Butler FK. **Antibiotics in Tactical Combat Casualty Care**. *Military Medicine*, 168:911-4, 2003.

SCOPE OF PRACTICE

RANGER FIRST RESPONDER (RFR) – A Ranger who has successfully completed the Ranger First Responder Course. RFRs conduct their scope of practice under the license of a medical director. Every Ranger is to be RFR qualified.

THE 8 "CRITICAL" RFR TASKS:

CARE UNDER FIRE

1) **C**ontain Scene and Assess Casualties
   - Return Fire and Secure Scene
   - Direct Casualties to Cover
   - Evaluate for Life Threatening Injuries
   - Triage – Immediate, Delayed, Minimal, Expectant
   - Call Medical Personnel for Assistance as Required

2) **R**apidly Identify and Control Massive Hemorrhage
   - Direct & Indirect Pressure
   - Tourniquet
   - Emergency Trauma Dressing

TACTICAL FIELD CARE

3) **I**nspect and Ensure Patent Airway
   - Open and Clear Airway
   - Nasopharyngeal Airway

4) **T**reat Life Threatening Torso Injuries
   - Occlusive Seal Dressing
   - Needle Decompression
   - Abdominal wound management

5) **I**nspect for Bleeding, Gain IV Access, Manage Shock
   - Head to Toe Blood Sweeps
   - 18 Gauge Saline Lock
   - IV Fluids when dictated by Shock
   - Prevent Hypothermia

6) **C**ontrol Pain and Prevent Infection
   - Combat Wound Pill Pack

CASEVAC

7) **A**id and Litter Team
   - Package and Prepare for Transfer
   - SKEDCO, Litters, Manual Carries

8) **L**eader Coordinated Evacuation
   - Casualty Precedence – Critical (Urgent), Priority, Routine
   - CASEVAC or MEDEVAC Coordination

SQUAD EMT – A non-medical MOS Ranger currently registered as an EMT-Basic/Intermediate by the Department of Transportation (DOT) and designated by the command to operate in this capacity. This individual functions as a bridge between the RFR and the Ranger Medic in respect to tactical and administrative trauma management. Squad EMTs conduct their scope of practice under the licensure of a medical director.

SPECIAL OPERATIONS COMBAT MEDIC ADVANCED TACTICAL PRACTITIONER (SOCM-ATP) – A Ranger Medic currently registered as an NREMT-Paramedic by the DOT and/or USSOCOM State-Paramedic (Advanced Tactical Practitioner) who has been awarded the identifier W1 (Special Operations Combat Medic) and has been approved by the unit Medical Director to function at this advanced level of care. A Ranger Medic can train and direct routine and emergency medical care, establish combat casualty collection points, conduct initial surgical and medical patient assessment and management, triage and provide advanced trauma management, and prepare patients for evacuation.

Routine garrison care includes assisting unit medical officers with daily sick call and requires advanced knowledge in common orthopedic problems, respiratory illnesses, gastrointestinal disorders, dermatological conditions, and environmental hazard illnesses. Ranger Medics train non-medical personnel on first responder skills and preventive medicine. Ranger Medics conduct their scope of practice under the licensure of a medical director and are not independent health care providers. Ranger Medics should always obtain medical director advice and supervision for all care provided. However, on rare occasions Ranger Medics may be required to operate relatively independently with only indirect supervision in remote, austere, or clandestine locations. In these cases, it is still extremely rare that a Ranger Medic will be unable to communicate by radio, phone, or computer.

STANDING ORDERS – Advanced life support interventions, which may be undertaken _before_ contacting an on-line medical control.

PROTOCOLS – Guidelines for out of hospital patient care. Only the portions of the guidelines, which are designated as "standing orders", may be undertaken before contacting an on-line medical director.

MEDICAL CONTROL / MEDICAL DIRECTOR / MEDICAL OFFICER – A licensed and credentialed medical provider, physician or physician assistant, who verbally, or in writing, states assumption of responsibility and liability and is available on-site or can be contacted through established communications. Medical care, procedures, and advanced life-saving activities will be routed through medical control in order to provide optimal care to all sick or injured Rangers. Medical Control will always be established, regardless of whether the scenario is a combat mission, a training exercise, or routine medical care. **Note that, ultimately, all medical care is conducted under the licensure of an assigned, attached, augmenting, or collocated physician.**

STANDING ORDERS AND PROTOCOLS

These standing orders and protocols are only to be used by Ranger Medics assigned to the 75th Ranger Regiment.

PURPOSE

The primary purpose of these protocols is to serve as a guideline for tactical and non-tactical pre-hospital trauma and medical care. Quality out-of-hospital care is the direct result of comprehensive education, accurate patient assessment, good judgment, and continuous quality improvement. All Ranger medical personnel are expected to know the Trauma Management Team Protocols and understand the reasoning behind their employment. Ranger Medics should not perform any step in a standing order or protocol if they have not been trained to perform the procedure or treatment in question. Emergency, trauma, and tactical medicine continues to evolve at a rapid pace. Accordingly, this document is subject to change as new information and guidelines become available and are accepted by the medical community.

STANDING ORDERS AND PROTOCOLS

These standing orders and protocols are ONLY for use by Ranger Medics while providing BLS, ACLS, PHTLS, TCCC, and TMEPs. Ranger Medics who are authorized to operate under the Trauma Management Team guidelines may not utilize these standing orders outside of their military employment. All Ranger Medics **must adhere** to the standards defined in these protocols. Revocation of privileges will be considered by the granting authority if these standards are violated.

COMMUNICATIONS

In a case where the Ranger Medic cannot contact Medical Control due to an acute time-sensitive injury or illness, a mass casualty scenario, or communication difficulties, all protocols become standing orders. Likewise, in the event that Medical Control cannot respond to the radio or telephone in a timely fashion required to provide optimal care to a patient, all protocols are considered standing orders. In the event that Medical Control was not contacted, and treatment protocols were carried out as standing orders, Medical Control will be contacted as soon as feasible following the incident and the medical record (SF 600 or Trauma SF 600) will be reviewed and countersigned by Medical Control. Retroactive approval for appropriate care will be provided through this process.

When communicating with medical control, a medical officer or a receiving facility, a verbal report will include the following essential elements:

1. **Provider** – name, unit, and call back phone number
2. **Patient** – name, unit, age, and gender
3. **Subjective** – findings to include chief complaint and brief history of event
4. **Objective** – findings to include mental status, vital signs, and physical exam
5. **Assessment** – to include differential diagnosis and level of urgency
6. **Plan** – to include treatment provided, patient response to treatment, and ETA

Provide patient status updates as dictated by patient status changes en route.

PATIENT CARE DOCUMENTATION

Patient care documentation is of paramount importance and should be performed for every patient encounter using a JTF Combat Casualty Card, a Trauma SF 600 Medical Record, or a SF 600 Medical Record.

RESUSCITATION CONSIDERATIONS

Resuscitation is not warranted in patients who have sustained obvious life-ending trauma, or patients with rigor mortis, decapitation, or decomposition. However, when reasonable, consider performing resuscitation efforts when this is your only patient. The perception of fellow Rangers and family members in this instance should be that every effort was made to sustain life. When possible, place "quick look" paddles or EKG leads to confirm asystole or an agonal rhythm in two leads and attach a copy of this strip to the medical record. Also note that, technically, only a medical officer can pronounce a patient as deceased.

GENERAL GUIDELINES FOR PROTOCOL USAGE

1. The patient history should not be obtained at the expense of the patient. Life-threatening problems detected during the primary assessment must be treated first.

2. Cardiac arrest due to trauma is not treated by medical cardiac arrest protocols. Trauma patients should be transported promptly to the previously coordinated Medical Treatment Facility with CPR, control of external hemorrhage, cervical spine immobilization, and other indicated procedures attempted en route.

3. In patients who require a saline lock or intravenous fluids, only two attempts at IV access should be attempted in the field. Intraosseous infusion should be considered for life-threatening emergencies. However, patient transport to definitive care **must not be delayed** for multiple attempts at IV access or advanced medical procedures.

4. Medics will verbally repeat all orders received and given prior to their initiation. It is preferable that medical personnel work as two-man Trauma Teams whenever practical.

NEVER HESITATE TO CONTACT A MEDICAL DIRECTOR AT ANY TIME FOR ASSISTANCE, QUESTIONS, CLARIFICATION, OR GUIDANCE.

CASUALTY ASSESSMENT AND MANAGEMENT

I. OVERVIEW:

ESTABLISH PRIORITIES

1. **Obtain situational awareness…then ensure scene security**.
2. **Control yourself…then take control of the situation**. *The senior medical person on the scene needs to control the resuscitation effort. All orders to team members need to come from one person,* ***the senior medical person in charge.***
3. Just remember, there are three groups of casualties that you may encounter. With the first group, no matter what you do, they will live. With the second group, no matter what you do, they may die. With the third group, if you do the right thing, at the right time, your treatment will be the difference between life and death. Focus your efforts on this third group.

TRIAGE CATEGORIES

o **Immediate** – casualties with high chances of survival who require life-saving surgical procedures or medical care
o **Delayed** – casualties who require surgery or medical care, but whose general condition permits a delay in treatment without unduly endangering the casualty
o **Minimal** – casualties who have relatively minor injuries or illnesses and can effectively care for themselves or be helped by non-medical personnel
o **Expectant** – casualties who have wounds that are so extensive that even if they were the sole casualty and had the benefit of optimal medical resource application, their survival would be unlikely

EVACUATION PRECEDENCES ("CPR")

o **Critical (Urgent)** – evacuate within 2 HOURS in order to save life, limb, or eyesight
o **Priority** – evacuate within 4 HOURS as critical and time sensitive medical care is not available locally, the patient's medical condition could deteriorate, and/or the patient cannot wait for routine evacuation.
o **Routine** – evacuate within 24 HOURS, as the patient's medical condition is not expected to deteriorate significantly while awaiting flight

PRIMARY SURVEY

During the primary survey, life-threatening conditions are identified and simultaneously managed. The primary survey consists of:

A - Airway Maintenance and C-spine Stabilization (situation dependent)
B - Breathing
C - Circulation with Control of Massive Hemorrhage (conducted first in combat setting)
D - Disability [mental status]
E - Exposure/Environmental Control [prevent hypothermia]

RESUSCITATION

Aggressive initial resuscitation should include hemorrhage control, airway establishment and protection, ventilation and oxygenation, IV fluid administration as needed, and hypothermia prevention. As resuscitative interventions are performed, the provider should reassess the patient for changes in status.

SECONDARY SURVEY

The secondary survey should consist of obtaining a brief history and conducting a complete head-to-toe evaluation of the trauma patient. This in-depth examination utilizes inspection, palpation, percussion, and auscultation, to evaluate the body in sections. Each section is examined individually.

TREATMENT PLAN

Initially, provide critical resuscitative efforts to resolve potential life-threatening injuries detected in the primary and secondary survey. Secondly, determine the patient disposition. Is the patient stable or unstable? What further diagnostic evaluation, operative intervention, or treatment is required? What level of medical care is needed? When does the patient need to be evacuated? All of these questions must be answered in a logical fashion in order to prioritize and mobilize the resources available.

II. THE PRIMARY SURVEY

The primary survey is broken down into five major areas: Airway and C-Spine Control, Breathing, Circulation, Disability, Exposure/Environment Control.

o *During combat operations, while operating under the auspices of Tactical Combat Casualty Care (TCCC), the primary survey is conducted as C-A-B-D-E instead of A-B-C-D-E.*

o *Hemorrhage control is the most common cause of preventable death in combat and thus takes priority over airway management in this environment.*

A. AIRWAY AND C-SPINE

The upper airway should be assessed to ascertain patency. Chin lift, jaw thrust, or suction may be helpful in reestablishing an airway. Specific attention should be directed toward the possibility of a cervical spine fracture. The patient's head and neck should never be hyper-extended or hyper-flexed to establish or maintain an airway. One should assume a c-spine fracture in any patient with an injury above the clavicle. Approximately fifteen percent of patients who have this type of injury will also have a c-spine injury. Quick assessment of Airway & Breathing can be observed by the patient's ability to communicate and mentate.

B. BREATHING

The patient's chest should be exposed and you should look for <u>symmetrical</u> movement of the chest wall. Conditions that often compromise ventilation include: MASSIVE HEMOTHORAX, TENSION PNEUMOTHORAX, OPEN PNEUMOTHORAX, and FLAIL CHEST.

C. CIRCULATION

Circulation is divided into two parts: Hemodynamic Status and Hemorrhage Control.

1. Hemodynamic Status

A formal blood pressure measurement **SHOULD NOT** be performed at this point in the primary survey. Important information can be rapidly obtained regarding perfusion and oxygenation from the level of consciousness, pulse, skin color, and capillary refill time. Decreased cerebral perfusion may result in an altered mental status. The patient's pulse is easily accessible, and if palpable, the systolic blood pressure in millimeters of mercury (mm HG) can be roughly determined as follows:

RADIAL PULSE:	**PRESSURE ≥ 80 mm Hg**
FEMORAL PULSE:	**PRESSURE ≥ 70 mm Hg**
CAROTID PULSE:	**PRESSURE ≥ 60 mm Hg**

Skin color and capillary refill will provide a rapid initial assessment of peripheral perfusion. Pink skin is a good sign versus the ominous sign of white or ashen, gray skin depicting hypovolemia. Pressure to the thumb nail or hypothenar eminence will cause the underlying tissue to blanch. In a normovolemic patient, the color returns to normal within two seconds. In the hypovolemic, poorly oxygenated patient and/or hypothermic patient this time period is extended or absent.

2. Hemorrhage Control (Conducted first in Combat Setting)

o **EXTERNAL HEMORRHAGE.** Exsanguinating external hemorrhage should be identified and controlled in the primary survey. Direct pressure, indirect pressure, elevation, tourniquets, hemostatic agents, and pressure dressings should be utilized to control bleeding. Note that tourniquets should be used as a primary adjunct for massive or arterial bleeding until controlled by dressings or hemostatic agents.

o **INTERNAL HEMORRHAGE.** Occult hemorrhage into the thoracic, abdominal, or pelvic region, or into the thigh surrounding a femur fracture, can account for significant blood loss. If an operating room is not immediately available, abdominal or lower extremity hemorrhage can be reduced by hemostatic agents, wound packing, ligation, and clamping.

Estimate of Fluid and Blood Requirements in Shock:				
	Class I	Class II	Class III	Class IV
Blood Loss (ml)	Up to 750	750-1500	1500-2000	> 2000
Blood Loss(%BV)	Up to 15%	15-30%	30-40%	> 40%
Pulse Rate	< 100	> 100	> 120	> 140
Blood Pressure	WNL	WNL	Decreased	Decreased
Pulse Pressure (mmHg)	WNL/increased	Decreased	Decreased	Decreased
Capillary Blanch Test	Normal	Positive	Positive	Positive
Respiratory Rate	14-20	20-30	30-40	> 35
Urine Output (mL/hr)	> 30	20-30	5-15	Negligible
CNS-Mental Status	Slightly anxious	Mildly anxious	Anxious/confused	Confused/lethargic
Fluid Replacement	Saline Lock	Saline Lock	Colloid / Blood	Colloid / Blood

D. DISABILITY (MENTAL STATUS)

A rapid neurologic evaluation should be utilized to determine the patient's pupillary size and response, as well as the level of consciousness (LOC). Pupils should be equally round and reactive to light. If the pupils are found to be sluggish or nonreactive to light with unilateral or bilateral dilation, one should suspect a head injury and/or inadequate brain perfusion. LOC can be described through either the AVPU or Glasgow Coma Scale (GCS) method:

AVPU:	A	ALERT
	V	Responds to **VERBAL** stimuli
	P	Responds to **PAINFUL** stimuli
	U	**UNRESPONSIVE** to stimuli

GCS: (15 point scale)	E	EYE OPENING	Spontaneous	4
			To speech	3
			To pain	2
			None	1
	V	VERBAL RESPONSE	Oriented	5
			Confused	4
			Inappropriate Words	3
			Incomprehensible Sounds	2
			None	1
	M	MOTOR RESPONSE	Obeys Commands	6
			Localizes Pain	5
			Withdraws (Normal Flexion)	4
			Decorticate (Abnormal Flexion)	3
			Decerebrate (Extension)	2
			None (Flaccid)	1

E. EXPOSURE / ENVIRONMENTAL CONTROL

The patient should be completely undressed (environment permitting) to facilitate thorough examination and assessment during the secondary survey. Strive to maintain the patient in a normothermic state. **Hypothermia prevention is as important as any other resuscitation effort.**

III. RESUSCITATION

Resuscitation includes oxygenation, intravenous access, and monitoring.

OXYGEN AND AIRWAY MANAGEMENT

Supplemental oxygen should be administered to all trauma patients in the form of a nonrebreather mask if available. A bag-valve-mask (BVM) should be readily available and used when needed. Definitive airways can be provided through cricothyroidotomy and endotracheal intubation. Endotracheal intubation must be *confirmed and documented* by at least three of the following methods: 1) visualization of the tube passing through cords, 2) endotracheal esophageal detector (Tube Check), 3) bilateral breath sounds and absence of epigastric sounds, 4) condensation inside the endotracheal tube, and 5) end-tidal carbon dioxide monitoring.

IV ACCESS

A minimum of two 18 gauge IV/saline locks should be started in all multiple trauma patients. The rate of fluid administration is determined by the patient's hemodynamic status and whether or not hemorrhage is controlled. Fluid resuscitation is assessed by improvement in physiologic parameters such as the ventilatory rate, pulse, blood pressure, and urinary output. Trauma patients should receive 1-2 peripheral IV access saline locks. Trauma patients who have **controlled bleeding** and a Systolic BP <90 mm Hg should receive Hextend until the Systolic BP is >90 mm Hg up to a maximum of 1000 ml. Trauma patients with controlled bleeding and a systolic blood pressure >90 mm Hg, or uncontrolled hemorrhage, should receive a saline lock only and fluids TKO. Note that the external jugular vein is considered a peripheral vein. When peripheral access is inaccessible after a minimum of two unsuccessful peripheral IV attempts, a sternal intraosseous "FAST-1" device can be performed on adults who require life-saving fluids and/or medications. When practical, use a permanent marker to label each IV bag with the time initiated and completed, medications placed in the bag, allergies to medications, and the number of IV bags received.

MONITORING

All patients followed for multiple trauma wounds should be continuously monitored for vital sign instability. Dysrhythmias are frequently associated with blunt chest trauma and should be treated in the same fashion as arrhythmias secondary to heart disease.

IV. The Secondary Survey

This survey should include a complete history, a head-to-toe physical examination, and a reassessment of vital signs.

HISTORY

A patient's pertinent past medical history must be obtained. A useful mnemonic is the word **"AMPLE"**.

> **A**llergies
> **M**edications and nutritional supplements
> **P**ast medical illnesses and injuries
> **L**ast meal
> **E**vents associated to the injury

PHYSICAL

The physical exam can be divided into eight parts: Head, Face, C-Spine and Neck, Chest, Abdomen, Perineum and Rectum, Musculoskeletal, and Neurological.

1. HEAD

The secondary survey begins with a detailed examination of the scalp and head looking for signs of significant injury to include edema, contusions, lacerations, foreign bodies, evidence of fracture, CSF leak, or hemotympanum. The eyes should be evaluated for visual acuity, pupillary size, external ocular muscle function, conjunctival and fundal hemorrhage, and contact lenses (remove before edema presents).

2. FACE

Maxillofacial trauma, ___unassociated with airway compromise and/or major hemorrhage___, should be treated after the patient is completely stabilized. If the patient has midface trauma, suspect a cribiform plate fracture. If intubation is required in this scenario then it should be performed orally and NOT via the nasal route.

3. C-SPINE/NECK

Suspect an unstable cervical spine injury in patients with blunt head or maxillofacial trauma and/or mechanism of injury (static-line or freefall jump incident, fastrope or rappelling incident, aircraft mishap, motor vehicle collision, blast injury, fall > 20 feet). An absence of neurological deficits does not rule out spinal injuries. A cervical spine injury should be presumed and the neck immobilized until cleared by a physician and/or radiographic evaluation. Cervical spine tenderness to palpation and spasm of the musculature of the neck can be associated with a cervical spine injury. The absence of neck pain and spasm in a patient who is neurologically intact is good evidence that a C-spine injury does not exist. However, it does not eliminate the need for radiographic cervical spine evaluation. Neck inspection, palpation, and auscultation should also be used to evaluate for subcutaneous emphysema, tracheal deviation, laryngeal fracture, and carotid artery injury. In the absence of hypovolemia, neck vein distension can be suggestive of a tension pneumothorax or cardiac tamponade.

4. CHEST

A complete inspection of the anterior and posterior aspect of the chest must be performed to exclude an open pneumothorax or flail segment. The entire chest wall (rib cage, sternum, clavicles, and posterior and axillary regions) should be palpated to reveal unsuspected fractures or costochondral separation. Auscultation should be utilized to evaluate for the alteration of breath sounds denoting a pneumothorax, tension pneumothorax, or hemothorax. Auscultation of distant heart sounds may be indicative of a cardiac tamponade. Percussion of hypertympanic sounds may indicate tension pneumothorax.

5. ABDOMEN

Any abdominal injury is potentially dangerous. Once identified, these injuries must be treated early and aggressively. The specific diagnosis is not as important as the fact that an abdominal injury exists which may require surgical intervention. Palpation, close observation, and frequent reevaluation of the abdomen are essential in the assessment and management of an intra-abdominal injury. In blunt trauma, the initial examination of the abdomen may be unremarkable. However, serial exams over time may reveal increasing signs of tenderness, rebound pain, guarding, and loss of bowel sounds.

6. RECTUM

A complete rectal examination in a trauma patient is essential and should include an evaluation for rectal wall integrity, prostate position, sphincter tone, and gross or occult blood.

7. EXTREMITIES

Extremities should be inspected for lacerations, contusions, and deformities. Palpation of bones (through rotational or three-point pressure) checking for tenderness, crepitation, or abnormal movements along the shaft, can help to identify non-displaced or occult fractures. Slight pressure **(NO PELVIC ROCK)** with the heels of the hand on the anterior superior iliac spines and on the symphysis pubis can identify pelvic fractures. Peripheral pulses should be assessed on all four extremities. The absence of a peripheral pulse distal to a fracture or dislocation mandates manipulation toward the position of function; if the pulse is still absent, transport immediately.

8. NEUROLOGICAL EXAMINATION

An in-depth neurological examination includes motor and sensory evaluation of each extremity, and continuous re-evaluation of the patient's level of consciousness and pupil size and response. Any evidence of loss of sensation, weakness, or paralysis suggests a major injury either to the spinal column or peripheral nervous system. Immobilization using a long board and a rigid cervical collar must be immediately established. These patients should be evacuated as soon as possible. Additionally, consider treating patient as a spinal cord injury if distracting injury and consistent with mechanism of injury.

V. REEVALUATION

Trauma patients require serial exams and reevaluation for changed or new signs and symptoms. Continuous observation, monitoring, vital sign assessment, and urinary output maintenance (an average of > 30cc/hour in the adult patient) is also imperative. As initial life-threatening injuries are managed, other equally life-threatening problems may develop. Less severe injuries or underlying medical problems may become evident. A high index of suspicion facilitates early diagnosis and management.

VI. SUMMARY

The injured Ranger must be rapidly and thoroughly evaluated. You must develop an outline of priorities for your patient. These priorities in combat include the primary survey which includes evaluation of circulation, airway and c-spine control, breathing, disability (mental status), and exposure/environment.

Resuscitation should proceed simultaneously with the primary survey. It includes the management of all life-threatening problems, the establishment of intravenous access, the placement of EKG monitoring equipment, and the administration of oxygen.

The secondary survey includes a total evaluation of the injured Ranger from head to toe. During your evaluation you reassess the ABC's and the interventions provided during the primary survey. Ensure to document your finding and interventions on a Trauma SF 600 or JTF Casualty Card.

TACTICAL COMBAT CASUALTY CARE (TCCC)

Trauma is the leading cause of death in the first four decades of life. Current protocols for civilian trauma care in the US are based on the Advanced Trauma Life Support (ATLS) course, which was initially conducted in 1978. Since that time, ATLS protocols have been accepted as the standard of care for the first hour of trauma management that is taught to both civilian and military providers. ATLS is a great approach in the civilian setting; however, it was never designed for combat application.

Historically, most combat-related deaths have occurred in close proximity to the point of injury prior to a casualty reaching an established medical treatment facility. The combat environment has many factors that affect medical care to include temperature and weather extremes, severe visual limitations, delays in treatment and evacuation, long evacuation distances, a lack of specialized providers and equipment near the scene, and the lethal implications of an opposing force. Thus, a modified approach to trauma management must be utilized while conducting combat operations.

Combat treatment protocols must be directed toward preventable combat death. COL Ron Bellamy researched how people die in ground combat and developed a list of causes of death that can be prevented on the battlefield.

How people die in combat	Preventable causes of death
KIA: 31% penetrating head trauma KIA: 25% surgically uncorrectable torso trauma KIA: 10% potentially correctable surgical trauma KIA: 9% exsanguination from extremity wounds KIA: 7% mutilating blast trauma KIA: 5% tension pneumothorax KIA: 1% airway problems DOW: 12% (mostly from infections and complications of shock)	60% Bleeding to death from extremity wounds 33% Tension pneumothorax 6% Airway obstruction (maxillofacial trauma)

The tactical environment and causes of combat death dictate a different approach for ensuring the best possible outcome for combat casualties while sustaining the primary focus of completing the mission. CAPT Frank Butler and LTC John Hagmann proposed such an approach in 1996. Their article, **"Tactical Combat Casualty Care in Special Operations"**, emphasized three major objectives and outlined three phases of care.

Objectives:	Phases of Care:
✓ **Treat the patient** ✓ **Prevent additional casualties** ✓ **Complete the mission**	1. **Care Under Fire** 2. **Tactical Field Care** 3. **Combat Casualty Evacuation (CASEVAC) Care**

Over the past decade, numerous military and civilian medical providers and multiple articles in the medical literature have endorsed the tenets of Tactical Combat Casualty Care (TCCC). TCCC was integrated into the 4th and subsequent editions of the Prehospital Trauma Life Support (PHTLS) textbook that is authored by the National Association of Emergency Medical Technicians in cooperation with the American College of Surgeons Committee on Trauma.

In 2002, the Committee on Tactical Combat Casualty Care (COTCCC) was established by the US Special Operations Command. Since then, the COTCCC has met on a regular basis in order to evaluate, modify, and make recommendations for TCCC protocols, procedures, and guidelines.

The following is a summary of the phases of care which includes updates from the COTCCC through 2006:

PHASES OF CARE:	
1. CARE UNDER FIRE	
Care provided at point of injury while under effective enemy fire, limited by equipment carried by provider. Major goals are to move casualty to safety, prevent further injury to the casualty and provider, stop life threatening external hemorrhage, and **gain and maintain fire superiority – the best medicine on the battlefield!**	➤ Return fire and take cover, direct casualty to return fire and take cover ➤ Keep yourself from getting shot and prevent additional wounds to casualty ➤ Self aid if able and buddy aid if available ➤ Treat life threatening external hemorrhage with a tourniquet ➤ If bleeding continues, also use a hemostatic agent and pressure dressing
2. TACTICAL FIELD CARE	
Care rendered once casualty is no longer under effective enemy fire or when conducting a mission without hostile fire. Do not attempt CPR on the battlefield for victims of blast or penetrating trauma who have no pulse, respirations, or other signs of life. Disarm casualties with altered mental status, place weapon on safe and clear, take radio away from casualty.	➤ **AIRWAY** • Chin-lift or jaw-thrust maneuver, recovery position, and nasopharyngeal airway for unconscious patients • Cricothyroidotomy for airway obstruction • No C-Spine immobilization for penetrating trauma ➤ **BREATHING** • If torso trauma and respiratory distress, presume tension pneumothorax and needle decompress • Treat sucking chest wounds with three-sided dressing during expiration, and monitor for tension pneumothorax • Administer chest tube when needed

> **CIRCULATION**
>   - Assess and control bleeding with tourniquet, hemostatic agent, pressure dressing
>   - Initiate 18-gauge saline lock (IV); use IO as required
>   - Controlled hemorrhage, no shock: **NO FLUIDS**
>   - Controlled hemorrhage, shock: **Hextend 500-1000cc**
>   - Uncontrolled hemorrhage, no shock: **NO FLUIDS**
>   - PO fluids permissible if conscious
> **ENVIRONMENT**
>   - Prevent hypothermia, minimize exposure, external warming devices, IVF warmers
> **WOUNDS**
>   - Inspect, dress, and check for additional wounds
> **FRACTURES**
>   - Check pulse, inspect, dress, splint, and recheck pulse
> **MEDICATIONS (Analgesia and Antibiotics)**
>   - **Oral Wound Pill Packs:** Mobic 15 mg, Tylenol 650 mg, Moxifloxacin 400 mg
>   - **OTFC:** Fentanyl lozenge 800 mcg
>   - **IV Pain Management:** Morphine 5 mg IV repeated every 10 minutes as needed for pain; Promethazine 25 mg IV for nausea and synergistic analgesic effect
>   - **IV Antibiotic:** Cefotetan 2g q12h or Ertapenem 1 g q24h
> **MONITOR**
>   - Vital signs and pulse oximetry
> **DOCUMENT**
>   - Casualty Card

3. COMBAT CASUALTY EVACUATION (CASEVAC)

The medical care provided during the evacuation of the casualty. Continue or initiate care as per previous phase. Pre-staged medical assets on CASEVAC should be utilized to provide the same or higher level of care rendered during the mission.

> **INITIATE AND CONTINUE CARE AS PER PREVIOUS PHASE**

> **EVALUATE AND REFINE CARE**
>   - Airway: Consider combitube or laryngeal mask airway or endotracheal intubation
>   - Breathing: Consider oxygen if available
>   - Circulation: Convert tourniquets as possible
>   - Environment: Adjust temperature in vehicle or aircraft

SECTION TWO

PART A

TRAUMA PROTOCOLS

Tactical Trauma Assessment

APPROVED
DATE: 01 OCT 06
Dr Kotwal
Dr Redman
Dr Cunningham
Dr Miles

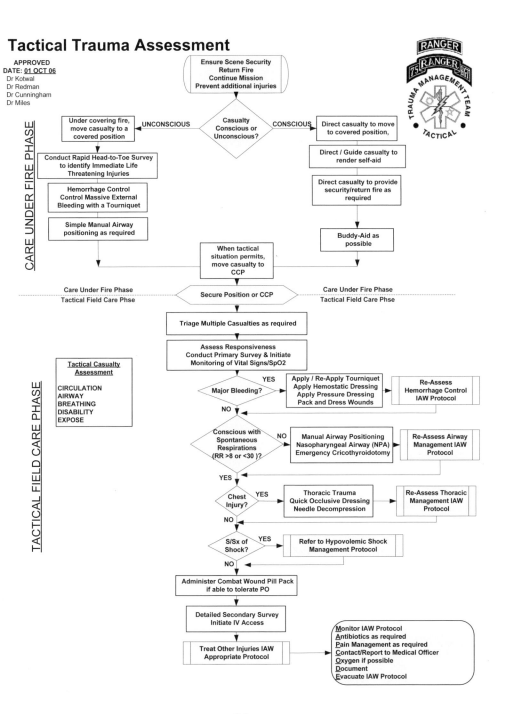

CARE UNDER FIRE PHASE

Ensure Scene Security
Return Fire
Continue Mission
Prevent additional injuries

Casualty Conscious or Unconscious?

UNCONSCIOUS →

Under covering fire, move casualty to a covered position

Conduct Rapid Head-to-Toe Survey to identify Immediate Life Threatening Injuries

Hemorrhage Control Control Massive External Bleeding with a Tourniquet

Simple Manual Airway positioning as required

← CONSCIOUS

Direct casualty to move to covered position,

Direct / Guide casualty to render self-aid

Direct casualty to provide security/return fire as required

Buddy-Aid as possible

When tactical situation permits, move casualty to CCP

Care Under Fire Phase
Tactical Field Care Phse

Secure Position or CCP

Care Under Fire Phase
Tactical Field Care Phse

TACTICAL FIELD CARE PHASE

Triage Multiple Casualties as required

Assess Responsiveness Conduct Primary Survey & Initiate Monitoring of Vital Signs/SpO2

Tactical Casualty Assessment

CIRCULATION
AIRWAY
BREATHING
DISABILITY
EXPOSE

Major Bleeding? — YES → Apply / Re-Apply Tourniquet Apply Hemostatic Dressing Apply Pressure Dressing Pack and Dress Wounds → Re-Assess Hemorrhage Control IAW Protocol

NO ↓

Conscious with Spontaneous Respirations (RR >8 or <30)? — NO → Manual Airway Positioning Nasopharyngeal Airway (NPA) Emergency Cricothyroidotomy → Re-Assess Airway Management IAW Protocol

YES ↓

Chest Injury? — YES → Thoracic Trauma Quick Occlusive Dressing Needle Decompression → Re-Assess Thoracic Management IAW Protocol

NO ↓

S/Sx of Shock? — YES → Refer to Hypovolemic Shock Management Protocol

NO ↓

Administer Combat Wound Pill Pack if able to tolerate PO

Detailed Secondary Survey Initiate IV Access

Treat Other Injuries IAW Appropriate Protocol →

Monitor IAW Protocol
Antibiotics as required
Pain Management as required
Contact/Report to Medical Officer
Oxygen if possible
Document
Evacuate IAW Protocol

RANGER
RANGER 75
TRAUMA MANAGEMENT TEAM
TACTICAL

2-1

Medical Patient Assessment Protocol

APPROVED
DATE: 01 OCT 06
Dr Kotwal
Dr Redman
Dr Cunningham
Dr Miles

RANGER
RANGER 75
TRAUMA MANAGEMENT TEAM
TACTICAL

AVPU Responsiveness Assessment

ALERT
VERBAL – Responds to verbal stimuli
PAIN – Responds to painful stimuli
UNCONSCIOUS – Does not respond to any stimuli

Glasgow Coma Scale

Eye	Spontaneous	4
Opening	To Voice	3
	To Pain	2
	None	1
Verbal	Oriented	5
Response	Confused	4
	Inappropriate Words	3
	Incomprehensible Words	2
	None	1
Motor	Obeys Commands	6
Response	Localizes Pain	5
	Withdraws (Pain)	4
	Flexion	3
	Extension	2
	None	1

Document as: E____ + V____ + M____ = ____

AMPLE Patient History
A – Allergies
M – Medications
P – Past Medical History
L – Last Meal
E – Events Associated

OPQRST Patient History
Chief Complaint
O – Onset
P – Provocation
Q – Quality
R – Radiation
S – Severity
T – Time

SOAP Format

S – Age/Sex
   Chief Complaint
   History of Present Illness
   Allergies
   Medications
   Past Medical History
   Past Surgical History
   Social History
O – Complete Vital Signs
   Physical Examination
A – Differential Diagnosis
P – Immediate Plan

Monitoring	Medications
Fluids	Diagnostics
Procedures	Referrals
Transport	

Flowchart

Indication for a Medical Patient Assessment
↓
Scene Secure? — NO → Ensure Scene Security or Refer to Tactical Assessment Protocol
↓ YES
Provider Precautions
↓
Primary Survey
A – Airway / C-Spine
B – Breathing
C – Circulation
D – Disability
E – Expose/Environment
↓
Detailed Assessment & Documentaton
Complete Vital Signs
SOAP Format
↓
Continuous Monitoring Required? — YES → Consider: Cardiac Monitoring, Pulsoximetry, Glucometry, IV Access
↓ NO
Focused Examination Based on Chief Complaints)
↓
Apply appropriate protocols based on Primary, Detailed and Focused Assessments
↓
Document all findings
↓
Monitor IAW Protocol
Antibiotics as required
Pain Management as required
Contact/Report to Medical Officer
Oxygen if possible
Document
Evacuate IAW Protocol

Normal Adult Vital Signs
Systolic Blood Pressure:
   Male: 120-140
   Female: 110-130
Pulse Rate: 60-80
Respiratory Rate: 12-20
Body Temperature: 98.6

Abnormal Finding: Eyes, Ears, Nose
Cerebral Spinal Fluid
Battle's Sign
Raccoon eyes
Pupil Inequality
Abnormal gaze
Doll's eye response

Abnormal Finding: Neck
Jugular vein distention
Tracheal deviation
Subcutaneous emphysema

Abnormal Finding: Chest & Breath Sounds
Retractions
Unequal excursion
Subcutaneous emphysema
Erythema
Paradoxical motion
Abnormal breath sounds
Rales
Rhonchi
Wheezing
Stridor
Kussmaul respirations
Cheyne-stokes pattern

Abnormal Finding: Abdominal
Pulsations
Guarding
Pain
Tenderness
Rebound tenderness
Masses
Absent bowel sounds

Signs of Extremity Vascular Compromise
Absent or diminshed pulse
Cool extremity
Slow or absent capillary refill
Cyanosis
Dislocation
Inappropriate Angles
Swelling
Discoloration

Airway Management Protocol

APPROVED
DATE: 01 OCT 06
Dr Kotwal
Dr Redman
Dr Cunningham
Dr Miles

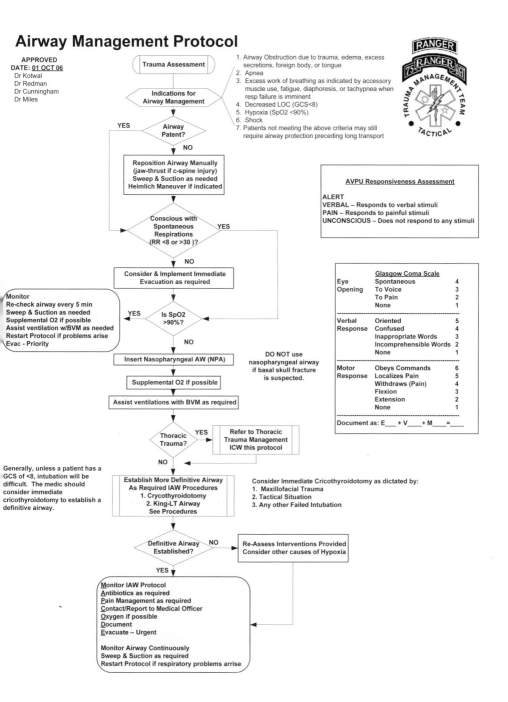

Trauma Assessment

Indications for Airway Management

1. Airway Obstruction due to trauma, edema, excess secretions, foreign body, or tongue
2. Apnea
3. Excess work of breathing as indicated by accessory muscle use, fatigue, diaphoresis, or tachypnea when resp failure is imminent
4. Decreased LOC (GCS<8)
5. Hypoxia (SpO2 <90%)
6. Shock
7. Patients not meeting the above criteria may still require airway protection preceding long transport

Airway Patent? — YES / NO

Reposition Airway Manually (jaw-thrust if c-spine injury) Sweep & Suction as needed Heimlich Maneuver if indicated

AVPU Responsiveness Assessment

ALERT
VERBAL – Responds to verbal stimuli
PAIN – Responds to painful stimuli
UNCONSCIOUS – Does not respond to any stimuli

Conscious with Spontaneous Respirations (RR <8 or >30)? — YES / NO

Consider & Implement Immediate Evacuation as required

Monitor
Re-check airway every 5 min
Sweep & Suction as needed
Supplemental O2 if possible
Assist ventilation w/BVM as needed
Restart Protocol if problems arise
Evac - Priority

Is SpO2 >90%? — YES / NO

Insert Nasopharyngeal AW (NPA)

DO NOT use nasopharyngeal airway if basal skull fracture is suspected.

Supplemental O2 if possible

Assist ventilations with BVM as required

	Glasgow Coma Scale	
Eye Opening	Spontaneous	4
	To Voice	3
	To Pain	2
	None	1
Verbal Response	Oriented	5
	Confused	4
	Inappropriate Words	3
	Incomprehensible Words	2
	None	1
Motor Response	Obeys Commands	6
	Localizes Pain	5
	Withdraws (Pain)	4
	Flexion	3
	Extension	2
	None	1

Document as: E____ + V____ + M____ = ____

Thoracic Trauma? — YES → **Refer to Thoracic Trauma Management ICW this protocol** / NO

Generally, unless a patient has a GCS of <8, intubation will be difficult. The medic should consider immediate cricothyroidotomy to establish a definitive airway.

Establish More Definitive Airway As Required IAW Procedures
1. Crycothyroidotomy
2. King-LT Airway
See Procedures

Consider Immediate Cricothyroidotomy as dictated by:
1. Maxillofacial Trauma
2. Tactical Situation
3. Any other Failed Intubation

Definitive Airway Established? — NO → **Re-Assess Interventions Provided Consider other causes of Hypoxia** / YES

Monitor IAW Protocol
Antibiotics as required
Pain Management as required
Contact/Report to Medical Officer
Oxygen if possible
Document
Evacuate – Urgent

Monitor Airway Continuously
Sweep & Suction as required
Restart Protocol if respiratory problems arrise

RANGER 75 RANGER
TRAUMA MANAGEMENT TEAM
TACTICAL

Surgical Cricothyroidotomy Procedure

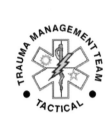

APPROVED
DATE: 01 OCT 06
Dr Kotwal
Dr Redman
Dr Cunningham
Dr Miles

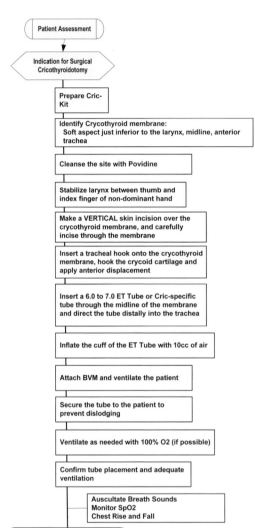

Patient Assessment

Indication for Surgical Cricothyroidotomy

Prepare Cric-Kit

Identify Crycothyroid membrane:
 Soft aspect just inferior to the larynx, midline, anterior trachea

Cleanse the site with Povidine

Stabilize larynx between thumb and index finger of non-dominant hand

Make a VERTICAL skin incision over the cryocothyroid membrane, and carefully incise through the membrane

Insert a tracheal hook onto the crycothyroid membrane, hook the crycoid cartilage and apply anterior displacement

Insert a 6.0 to 7.0 ET Tube or Cric-specific tube through the midline of the membrane and direct the tube distally into the trachea

Inflate the cuff of the ET Tube with 10cc of air

Attach BVM and ventilate the patient

Secure the tube to the patient to prevent dislodging

Ventilate as needed with 100% O2 (if possible)

Confirm tube placement and adequate ventilation

Auscultate Breath Sounds
Monitor SpO2
Chest Rise and Fall

Monitor Continuously
Antibiotics as required
Pain Management as required
Contact/Report to Medical Officer
Oxygen if possible
Document
Evacuate IAW Protocol

Ensure adequate ventilation with BVM (12 to 20 breaths per minute)

EQUIPMENT NEEDED:
 - Scalpel, Sz 10
 - Tracheal Hook
 - Povidine Solution/Swab
 - Gloves
 - Sterile 4X4 Sponge
 - 7.0mm ET Tube
 - Bag-Valve-Mask (BVM)

DOCUMENTATION:
 - ABC's
 - Detailed Assessment
 - Vital Signs
 - SpO2
 - Glasgow Coma Scale
 - Tube Check Results
 - Lung Sounds
 - Absence of Epigastric Sonds
 - Skin Color
 - Complications Encountered

	Glasgow Coma Scale	
Eye	Spontaneous	4
Opening	To Voice	3
	To Pain	2
	None	1
Verbal	Oriented	5
Response	Confused	4
	Inappropriate Words	3
	Incomprehensible Words	2
	None	1
Motor	Obeys Commands	6
Response	Localizes Pain	5
	Withdraws (Pain)	4
	Flexion	3
	Extension	2
	None	1

Document as: E___ + V____ + M____ = ____

1. Maintain strict C-Spine precautions if potential for C-Spine Injury exists.
2. Anytime the patient goes 30 seconds without ventilation, stop the procedure and hyperventilate for 30-60 seconds before procedure is re-attempted.

King-LT D Supralaryngeal Airway Insertion Procedure

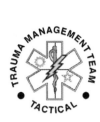

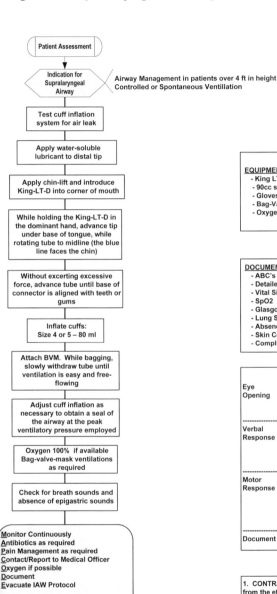

Patient Assessment

↓

Indication for Supralaryngeal Airway → Airway Management in patients over 4 ft in height
Controlled or Spontaneous Ventillation

↓

Test cuff inflation system for air leak

↓

Apply water-soluble lubricant to distal tip

↓

Apply chin-lift and introduce King-LT-D into corner of mouth

↓

While holding the King-LT-D in the dominant hand, advance tip under base of tongue, while rotating tube to midline (the blue line faces the chin)

↓

Without excerting excessive force, advance tube until base of connector is aligned with teeth or gums

↓

Inflate cuffs: Size 4 or 5 – 80 ml

↓

Attach BVM. While bagging, slowly withdraw tube until ventilation is easy and free-flowing

↓

Adjust cuff inflation as necessary to obtain a seal of the airway at the peak ventilatory pressure employed

↓

Oxygen 100% if available
Bag-valve-mask ventilations as required

↓

Check for breath sounds and absence of epigastric sounds

↓

Monitor Continuously
Antibiotics as required
Pain Management as required
Contact/Report to Medical Officer
Oxygen if possible
Document
Evacuate IAW Protocol

Ensure adequate ventilation with BVM (12 to 20 breaths per minute)

APPROVED
DATE: 01 OCT 06
Dr Kotwal
Dr Redman
Dr Cunningham
Dr Miles

EQUIPMENT NEEDED:
- King LT-D Airway Device (siz 4 or 5)
- 90cc syringe (accompanying)
- Gloves
- Bag-Valve-Mask (BVM)
- Oxygen if available

DOCUMENTATION:
- ABC's
- Detailed Assessment
- Vital Signs
- SpO2
- Glasgow Coma Scale
- Lung Sounds
- Absence of Epigastric Sonds
- Skin Color
- Complications Encountered

Glasgow Coma Scale

Eye Opening	Spontaneous	4
	To Voice	3
	To Pain	2
	None	1
Verbal Response	Oriented	5
	Confused	4
	Inappropriate Words	3
	Incomprehensible Words	2
	None	1
Motor Response	Obeys Commands	6
	Localizes Pain	5
	Withdraws (Pain)	4
	Flexion	3
	Extension	2
	None	1

Document as: E___ + V____ + M____ = ____

1. CONTRAINDICATION: The King-LT-D does not protect the airway from the effects of reguritation or aspiration. Be prepared to suction as needed.
2. REMOVAL:
   a. Suction above the cuff in the oral cavity if indicated
   b. Fully deflate both cuffs before removal of the device
   c. Remove the King LT-D when protective reflexes have returned

Orotracheal Intubation Procedure

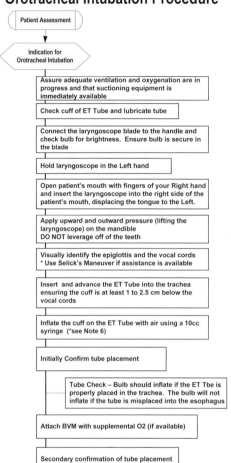

Patient Assessment

▼

Indication for
Orotracheal Intubation

Assure adequate ventilation and oxygenation are in progress and that suctioning equipment is immediately available

Check cuff of ET Tube and lubricate tube

Connect the laryngoscope blade to the handle and check bulb for brightness. Ensure bulb is secure in the blade

Hold laryngoscope in the Left hand

Open patient's mouth with fingers of your Right hand and insert the laryngoscope into the right side of the patient's mouth, displacing the tongue to the Left.

Apply upward and outward pressure (lifting the laryngoscope) on the mandible
DO NOT leverage off of the teeth

Visually identify the epiglottis and the vocal cords
* Use Selick's Maneuver if assistance is available

Insert and advance the ET Tube into the trachea ensuring the cuff is at least 1 to 2.5 cm below the vocal cords

Inflate the cuff on the ET Tube with air using a 10cc syringe (*see Note 6)

Initially Confirm tube placement

Tube Check – Bulb should inflate if the ET Tbe is properly placed in the trachea. The bulb will not inflate if the tube is misplaced into the esophagus

Attach BVM with supplemental O2 (if available)

Secondary confirmation of tube placement

Auscultation – Bilateral breath sounds should be heard upon inhalation and/or squeezing of the BVM or epigastric sounds

Secure the Tube

Monitor Continuously
Antibiotics as required
Pain Management as required
Contact/Report to Medical Officer
Oxygen if possible
Document
Evacuate IAW Protocol

Ensure adequate ventilation with BVM
(12 to 20 breaths per minute)

TRAUMA MANAGEMENT TEAM TACTICAL

APPROVED
DATE: 01 OCT 06
Dr Kotwal
Dr Redman
Dr Cunningham
Dr Miles

EQUIPMENT NEEDED:
- Laryngoscope
- Miller and Macintosh Blades
- ET Tube (7.0 or 7.5mm)
- Suction (Manual or Mechanical)
- Oxygen Source (if available)
- Bag-Valve-Mask (BVM)
- Stylet
- Stethoscope
- Syringe, 10cc
- Lubricant (Water Soluble)
- Tube Check Bulb
- Pulsoximeter
- Gloves
- Tape

DOCUMENTATION:
- ABC's
- Detailed Assessment
- Vital Signs
- SpO2
- Glasgow Coma Scale
- Tube Check Results
- Lung Sounds
- Absence of Epigastric Sonds
- Skin Color
- Teeth to ET Tube Tip depth
- Complications Encountered

	Glasgow Coma Scale	
Eye Opening	Spontaneous	4
	To Voice	3
	To Pain	2
	None	1
Verbal Response	Oriented	5
	Confused	4
	Inappropriate Words	3
	Incomprehensible Words	2
	None	1
Motor Response	Obeys Commands	6
	Localizes Pain	5
	Withdraws (Pain)	4
	Flexion	3
	Extension	2
	None	1

Document as: E___ + V___ + M___ = ____

1. Maintain strict C-Spine precautions if potential for C-Spine Injury exists.
2. Avoid applying pressure on the teeth or lips. Never use a prying motion.
3. anytime the patient goes 30 seconds without ventilation, stop the procedure and hyperventilate for 30-60 seconds before procedure is re-attempted.
4. Intubation is to be only attempted twice. After two unsuccessful attempts are made, transition to a surgical cricothyroidotomy.
5. If assistance is available, use Selick's maneuver to assist visualization of epiglottis and vocal cords.
6. Inflate with 10cc of normal saline OR only 5cc of air for high altitude environment or high altitude aeromedical evacuation.

Hemorrhage Management Protocol

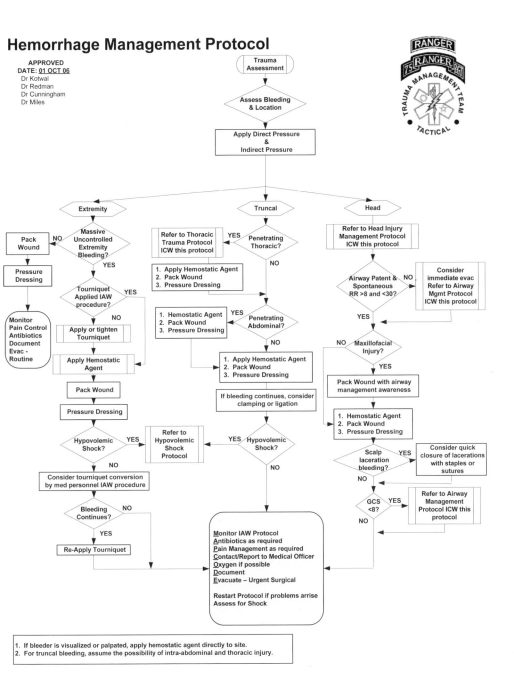

APPROVED
DATE: 01 OCT 06
Dr Kotwal
Dr Redman
Dr Cunningham
Dr Miles

Trauma Assessment

Assess Bleeding & Location

Apply Direct Pressure & Indirect Pressure

Extremity

Massive Uncontrolled Extremity Bleeding?

Pack Wound — NO

Pressure Dressing

Monitor
Pain Control
Antibiotics
Document
Evac - Routine

YES

Tourniquet Applied IAW procedure? — YES

NO

Apply or tighten Tourniquet

Apply Hemostatic Agent

Pack Wound

Pressure Dressing

Hypovolemic Shock? — YES — Refer to Hypovolemic Shock Protocol

NO

Consider tourniquet conversion by med personnel IAW procedure

Bleeding Continues? — NO

YES

Re-Apply Tourniquet

Truncal

Refer to Thoracic Trauma Protocol ICW this protocol — YES — Penetrating Thoracic?

NO

1. Apply Hemostatic Agent
2. Pack Wound
3. Pressure Dressing

1. Hemostatic Agent
2. Pack Wound
3. Pressure Dressing — YES — Penetrating Abdominal?

NO

1. Apply Hemostatic Agent
2. Pack Wound
3. Pressure Dressing

If bleeding continues, consider clamping or ligation

Hypovolemic Shock? — YES

NO

Head

Refer to Head Injury Management Protocol ICW this protocol

Airway Patent & Spontaneous RR >8 and <30? — NO — Consider immediate evac Refer to Airway Mgmt Protocol ICW this protocol

YES

NO — Maxillofacial Injury?

YES

Pack Wound with airway management awareness

1. Hemostatic Agent
2. Pack Wound
3. Pressure Dressing

Scalp laceration bleeding? — YES — Consider quick closure of lacerations with staples or sutures

NO

GCS <8? — YES — Refer to Airway Management Protocol ICW this protocol

NO

Monitor IAW Protocol
Antibiotics as required
Pain Management as required
Contact/Report to Medical Officer
Oxygen if possible
Document
Evacuate – Urgent Surgical

Restart Protocol if problems arrise
Assess for Shock

1. If bleeder is visualized or palpated, apply hemostatic agent directly to site.
2. For truncal bleeding, assume the possibility of intra-abdominal and thoracic injury.

Tourniquet Application Procedure

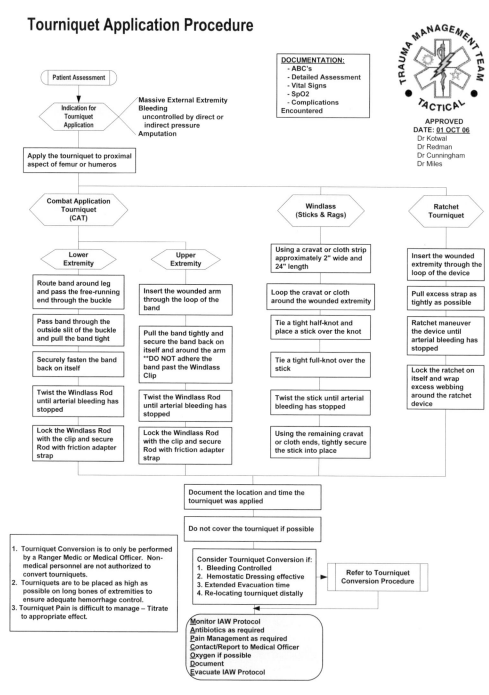

Patient Assessment

Indication for Tourniquet Application

Massive External Extremity Bleeding
uncontrolled by direct or indirect pressure
Amputation

Apply the tourniquet to proximal aspect of femur or humeros

DOCUMENTATION:
- ABC's
- Detailed Assessment
- Vital Signs
- SpO2
- Complications Encountered

Combat Application Tourniquet (CAT)

Windlass (Sticks & Rags)

Ratchet Tourniquet

Combat Application Tourniquet (CAT)

Lower Extremity

Route band around leg and pass the free-running end through the buckle

Pass band through the outside slit of the buckle and pull the band tight

Securely fasten the band back on itself

Twist the Windlass Rod until arterial bleeding has stopped

Lock the Windlass Rod with the clip and secure Rod with friction adapter strap

Upper Extremity

Insert the wounded arm through the loop of the band

Pull the band tightly and secure the band back on itself and around the arm **DO NOT adhere the band past the Windlass Clip

Twist the Windlass Rod until arterial bleeding has stopped

Lock the Windlass Rod with the clip and secure Rod with friction adapter strap

Windlass (Sticks & Rags)

Using a cravat or cloth strip approximately 2" wide and 24" length

Loop the cravat or cloth around the wounded extremity

Tie a tight half-knot and place a stick over the knot

Tie a tight full-knot over the stick

Twist the stick until arterial bleeding has stopped

Using the remaining cravat or cloth ends, tightly secure the stick into place

Ratchet Tourniquet

Insert the wounded extremity through the loop of the device

Pull excess strap as tightly as possible

Ratchet maneuver the device until arterial bleeding has stopped

Lock the ratchet on itself and wrap excess webbing around the ratchet device

---

Document the location and time the tourniquet was applied

Do not cover the tourniquet if possible

1. Tourniquet Conversion is to only be performed by a Ranger Medic or Medical Officer. Non-medical personnel are not authorized to convert tourniquets.
2. Tourniquets are to be placed as high as possible on long bones of extremities to ensure adequate hemorrhage control.
3. Tourniquet Pain is difficult to manage – Titrate to appropriate effect.

Consider Tourniquet Conversion if:
1. Bleeding Controlled
2. Hemostatic Dressing effective
3. Extended Evacuation time
4. Re-locating tourniquet distally

Refer to Tourniquet Conversion Procedure

Monitor IAW Protocol
Antibiotics as required
Pain Management as required
Contact/Report to Medical Officer
Oxygen if possible
Document
Evacuate IAW Protocol

Hemostatic Agent Application Procedure

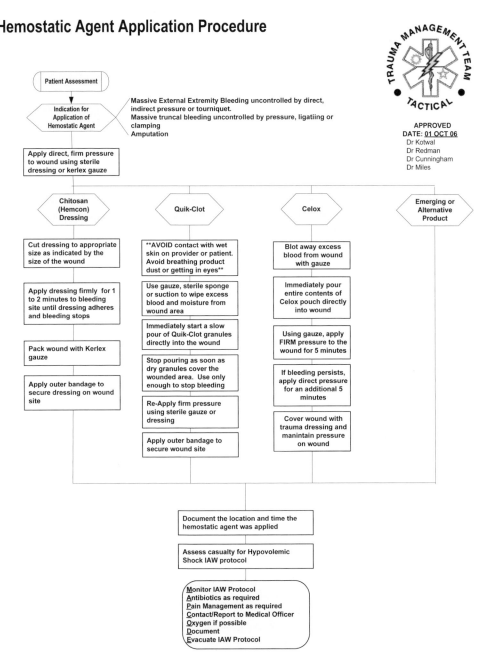

Patient Assessment

Indication for Application of Hemostatic Agent

Massive External Extremity Bleeding uncontrolled by direct, indirect pressure or tourniquet.
Massive truncal bleeding uncontrolled by pressure, ligatiing or clamping
Amputation

APPROVED
DATE: 01 OCT 06
Dr Kotwal
Dr Redman
Dr Cunningham
Dr Miles

Apply direct, firm pressure to wound using sterile dressing or kerlex gauze

Chitosan (Hemcon) Dressing

Cut dressing to appropriate size as indicated by the size of the wound

Apply dressing firmly for 1 to 2 minutes to bleeding site until dressing adheres and bleeding stops

Pack wound with Kerlex gauze

Apply outer bandage to secure dressing on wound site

Quik-Clot

AVOID contact with wet skin on provider or patient. Avoid breathing product dust or getting in eyes

Use gauze, sterile sponge or suction to wipe excess blood and moisture from wound area

Immediately start a slow pour of Quik-Clot granules directly into the wound

Stop pouring as soon as dry granules cover the wounded area. Use only enough to stop bleeding

Re-Apply firm pressure using sterile gauze or dressing

Apply outer bandage to secure wound site

Celox

Blot away excess blood from wound with gauze

Immediately pour entire contents of Celox pouch directly into wound

Using gauze, apply FIRM pressure to the wound for 5 minutes

If bleeding persists, apply direct pressure for an additional 5 minutes

Cover wound with trauma dressing and manintain pressure on wound

Emerging or Alternative Product

Document the location and time the hemostatic agent was applied

Assess casualty for Hypovolemic Shock IAW protocol

Monitor IAW Protocol
Antibiotics as required
Pain Management as required
Contact/Report to Medical Officer
Oxygen if possible
Document
Evacuate IAW Protocol

Tourniquet Conversion Procedure

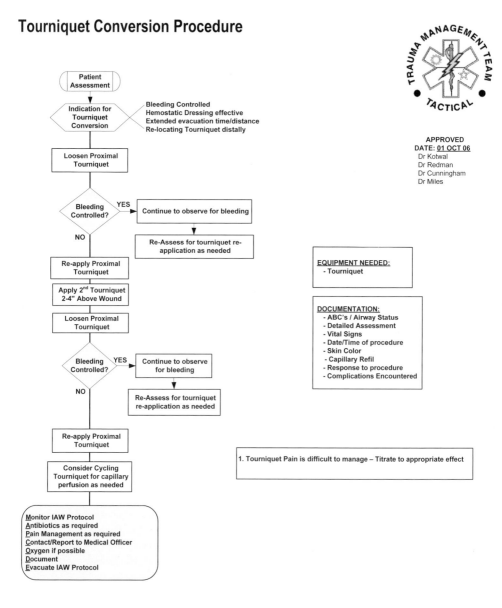

Patient Assessment

Indication for Tourniquet Conversion
- Bleeding Controlled
- Hemostatic Dressing effective
- Extended evacuation time/distance
- Re-locating Tourniquet distally

Loosen Proximal Tourniquet

Bleeding Controlled?
— YES → Continue to observe for bleeding → Re-Assess for tourniquet re-application as needed
— NO

Re-apply Proximal Tourniquet

Apply 2nd Tourniquet 2-4" Above Wound

Loosen Proximal Tourniquet

Bleeding Controlled?
— YES → Continue to observe for bleeding → Re-Assess for tourniquet re-application as needed
— NO

Re-apply Proximal Tourniquet

Consider Cycling Tourniquet for capillary perfusion as needed

Monitor IAW Protocol
Antibiotics as required
Pain Management as required
Contact/Report to Medical Officer
Oxygen if possible
Document
Evacuate IAW Protocol

TRAUMA MANAGEMENT TEAM
TACTICAL

APPROVED
DATE: 01 OCT 06
Dr Kotwal
Dr Redman
Dr Cunningham
Dr Miles

EQUIPMENT NEEDED:
- Tourniquet

DOCUMENTATION:
- ABC's / Airway Status
- Detailed Assessment
- Vital Signs
- Date/Time of procedure
- Skin Color
- Capillary Refil
- Response to procedure
- Complications Encountered

1. Tourniquet Pain is difficult to manage – Titrate to appropriate effect

Thoracic Trauma Management Protocol

APPROVED
DATE: 01 OCT 06
Dr Kotwal
Dr Redman
Dr Cunningham
Dr Miles

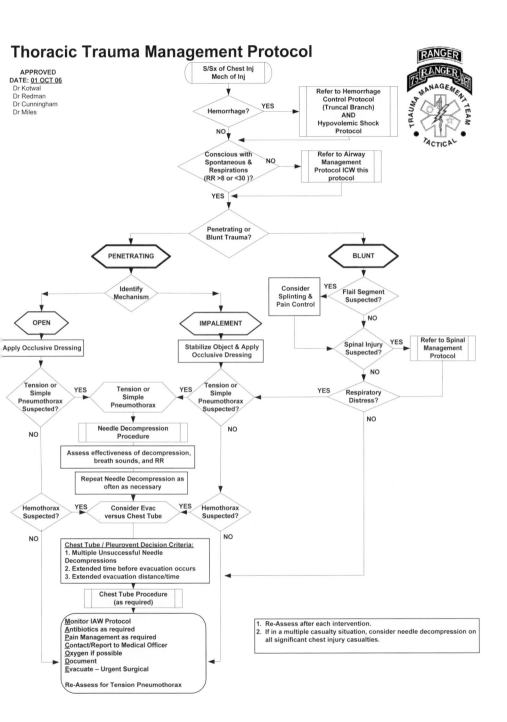

Needle Chest Decompression Procedure

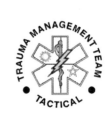

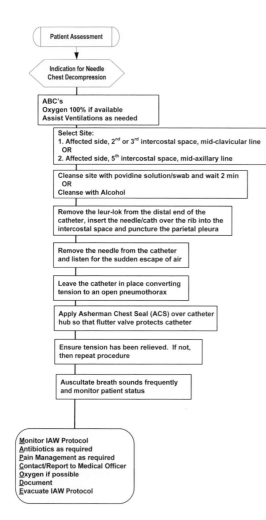

Patient Assessment

Indication for Needle
Chest Decompression

ABC's
Oxygen 100% if available
Assist Ventilations as needed

Select Site:
1. Affected side, 2nd or 3rd intercostal space, mid-clavicular line
   OR
2. Affected side, 5th intercostal space, mid-axillary line

Cleanse site with povidine solution/swab and wait 2 min
OR
Cleanse with Alcohol

Remove the leur-lok from the distal end of the catheter, insert the needle/cath over the rib into the intercostal space and puncture the parietal pleura

Remove the needle from the catheter and listen for the sudden escape of air

Leave the catheter in place converting tension to an open pneumothorax

Apply Asherman Chest Seal (ACS) over catheter hub so that flutter valve protects catheter

Ensure tension has been relieved. If not, then repeat procedure

Auscultate breath sounds frequently and monitor patient status

Monitor IAW Protocol
Antibiotics as required
Pain Management as required
Contact/Report to Medical Officer
Oxygen if possible
Document
Evacuate IAW Protocol

APPROVED
DATE: <u>01 OCT 06</u>
Dr Kotwal
Dr Redman
Dr Cunningham
Dr Miles

<u>EQUIPMENT NEEDED:</u>
- 10G to 14G 2.5" to 3" Needle with catheter
- Povidine Solution/swab
- Asherman Chest Seal

<u>DOCUMENTATION:</u>
- ABC's / Airway Status
- Detailed Assessment
- Vital Signs
- SpO2
- Lung Sounds before and after decompression
- Chest rise/excursion
- Skin Color
- Capillary refill
- Response to treatment
- Complications Encountered

1. The provider will make determination on site selection based on injury pattern and overall patient condition.
2. If using, povidine-iodine, wait 2 min before continuing with procedure

Chest Tube Insertion Procedure

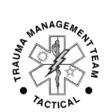

TRAUMA MANAGEMENT TEAM
TACTICAL

APPROVED
DATE: <u>01 OCT 06</u>
Dr Kotwal
Dr Redman
Dr Cunningham
Dr Miles

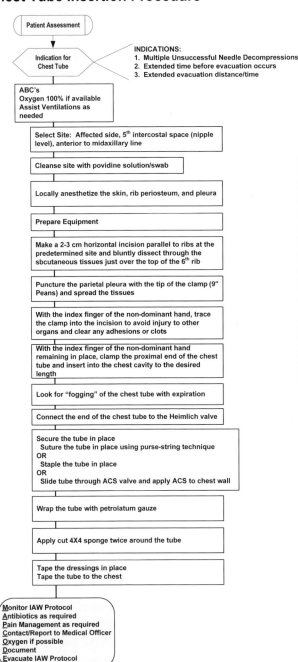

INDICATIONS:
1. Multiple Unsuccessful Needle Decompressions
2. Extended time before evacuation occurs
3. Extended evacuation distance/time

Patient Assessment

Indication for Chest Tube

ABC's
Oxygen 100% if available
Assist Ventilations as needed

Select Site: Affected side, 5th intercostal space (nipple level), anterior to midaxillary line

Cleanse site with povidine solution/swab

Locally anesthetize the skin, rib periosteum, and pleura

Prepare Equipment

Make a 2-3 cm horizontal incision parallel to ribs at the predetermined site and bluntly dissect through the sbcutaneous tissues just over the top of the 6th rib

Puncture the parietal pleura with the tip of the clamp (9" Peans) and spread the tissues

With the index finger of the non-dominant hand, trace the clamp into the incision to avoid injury to other organs and clear any adhesions or clots

With the index finger of the non-dominant hand remaining in place, clamp the proximal end of the chest tube and insert into the chest cavity to the desired length

Look for "fogging" of the chest tube with expiration

Connect the end of the chest tube to the Heimlich valve

Secure the tube in place
 Suture the tube in place using purse-string technique
OR
 Staple the tube in place
OR
 Slide tube through ACS valve and apply ACS to chest wall

Wrap the tube with petrolatum gauze

Apply cut 4X4 sponge twice around the tube

Tape the dressings in place
Tape the tube to the chest

Monitor IAW Protocol
Antibiotics as required
Pain Management as required
Contact/Report to Medical Officer
Oxygen if possible
Document
Evacuate IAW Protocol

EQUIPMENT NEEDED:
- 9" Peans Forceps (clamp)
- 1-0 Armed Suture
- Povidine Solution/swabs
- Scalpel, #10
- 36 Fr to 38 Fr Chest Tube
- Heimich Valve
- Sterile 4X4 Sponges
- Petrolatum Gauze
- 18G Needle
- Syringe, 10cc
- Chux
- Lidocain Inj, 1%
- Tape, 2"
- Sterile Gloves

DOCUMENTATION:
- ABC's / Airway Status
- Detailed Assessment
- Vital Signs
- SpO2
- Lung Sounds before and after tube insertion
- Chest rise/excursion
- Skin Color
- Capillary refill
- Response to treatment
- Complications Encountered

Hypovolemic Shock Management Protocol

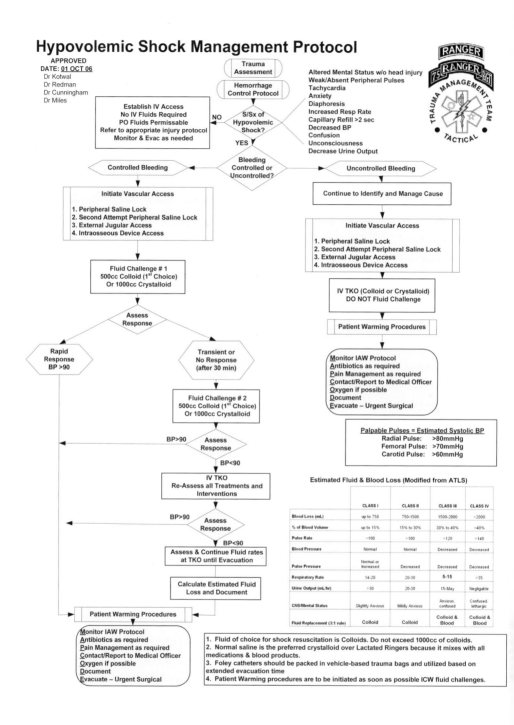

APPROVED
DATE: 01 OCT 06
Dr Kotwal
Dr Redman
Dr Cunningham
Dr Miles

Trauma Assessment

Hemorrhage Control Protocol

S/Sx of Hypovolemic Shock?

Altered Mental Status w/o head injury
Weak/Absent Peripheral Pulses
Tachycardia
Anxiety
Diaphoresis
Increased Resp Rate
Capillary Refill >2 sec
Decreased BP
Confusion
Unconsciousness
Decrease Urine Output

NO →
Establish IV Access
No IV Fluids Required
PO Fluids Permissable
Refer to appropriate injury protocol
Monitor & Evac as needed

YES ↓

Bleeding Controlled or Uncontrolled?

Controlled Bleeding

Initiate Vascular Access

1. Peripheral Saline Lock
2. Second Attempt Peripheral Saline Lock
3. External Jugular Access
4. Intraosseous Device Access

Fluid Challenge # 1
500cc Colloid (1st Choice)
Or 1000cc Crystalloid

Assess Response

Rapid Response BP >90

Transient or No Response (after 30 min)

Fluid Challenge # 2
500cc Colloid (1st Choice)
Or 1000cc Crystalloid

BP>90 ← Assess Response

BP<90 ↓

IV TKO
Re-Assess all Treatments and Interventions

BP>90 ← Assess Response

BP<90 ↓

Assess & Continue Fluid rates at TKO until Evacuation

Calculate Estimated Fluid Loss and Document

Patient Warming Procedures

Monitor IAW Protocol
Antibiotics as required
Pain Management as required
Contact/Report to Medical Officer
Oxygen if possible
Document
Evacuate – Urgent Surgical

Uncontrolled Bleeding

Continue to Identify and Manage Cause

Initiate Vascular Access

1. Peripheral Saline Lock
2. Second Attempt Peripheral Saline Lock
3. External Jugular Access
4. Intraosseous Device Access

IV TKO (Colloid or Crystalloid)
DO NOT Fluid Challenge

Patient Warming Procedures

Monitor IAW Protocol
Antibiotics as required
Pain Management as required
Contact/Report to Medical Officer
Oxygen if possible
Document
Evacuate – Urgent Surgical

Palpable Pulses = Estimated Systolic BP
Radial Pulse: >80mmHg
Femoral Pulse: >70mmHg
Carotid Pulse: >60mmHg

Estimated Fluid & Blood Loss (Modified from ATLS)

	CLASS I	CLASS II	CLASS III	CLASS IV
Blood Loss (mL)	up to 750	750-1500	1500-2000	>2000
% of Blood Volume	up to 15%	15% to 30%	30% to 40%	>40%
Pulse Rate	<100	>100	>120	>140
Blood Pressure	Normal	Normal	Decreased	Decreased
Pulse Pressure	Normal or Increased	Decreased	Decreased	Decreased
Respiratory Rate	14-20	20-30	5-15	>35
Urine Output (mL/hr)	>30	20-30	15-May	Negligable
CNS/Mental Status	Slightly Anxious	Mildly Anxious	Anxious, confused	Confused, lethargic
Fluid Replacement (3:1 rule)	Colloid	Colloid	Colloid & Blood	Colloid & Blood

1. Fluid of choice for shock resuscitation is Colloids. Do not exceed 1000cc of colloids.
2. Normal saline is the preferred crystalloid over Lactated Ringers because it mixes with all medications & blood products.
3. Foley catheters should be packed in vehicle-based trauma bags and utilized based on extended evacuation time
4. Patient Warming procedures are to be initiated as soon as possible ICW fluid challenges.

Saline Lock & Intravenous Access Procedure

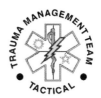

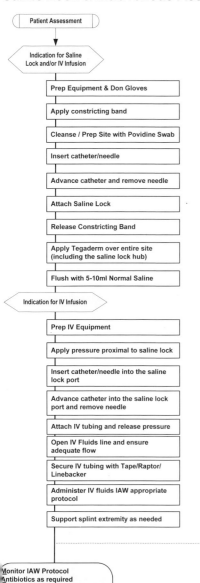

EQUIPMENT NEEDED:
- Constricting Band
- Povidine-Iodine Swab
- 2 X 18-G IV Catheter/Needle
- 10 cc Syringe
- Saline Lock
- Tegaderm (at least 2.5" X 2.5")
- IV Tubing (10 gtts/ml)
- Raptor/Linebacker IV securing device
- Tape, 2"
- Appropriate IV Fluids
- Gloves

DOCUMENTATION:
- ABC's
- Detailed Assessment
- Vital Signs
- SpO2
- IV Site
- IV Gauge
- Date/Time Started
- Fluids Infused / rate
- Complications Encountered

IV Drip Rates

* Hours To Deliver 1000 mL	ml per hour	10 Drops per ml. Drops Per Minute (DPM)	15 Drops per ml. Drops Per Minute (DPM)	20 Drops per ml. Drops Per Minute (DPM)	60 Drops per ml. Drops Per Minute (DPM)
Fractions are rounded to closest number, except where shown.	10	1.7 DPM	2.5 DPM	3 DPM	10 DPM
	30	5 DPM	7.5 DPM	10 DPM	30 DPM
	50	8 DPM	12.5 DPM	17 DPM	50 DPM
	70	12 DPM	17.5 DPM	23 DPM	70 DPM
	90	15 DPM	22.5 DPM	30 DPM	90 DPM
* 8 Hours	125	20.8 DPM	31 DPM	42 DPM	
	175	29 DPM	43.8 DPM	58 DPM	
	250	41.6 DPM	62.5 DPM	83 DPM	

Indication rapid removal of IV from saline Lock

Unsecure IV Tubing from PT and turn off the IV flow

Gently remove the IV tubing catheter from the saline lock
** DO NOT REMOVE THE SALINE LOCK**

Discard IV Bag/Tubing as appropriate

External Jugular Intravenous Cannulation Procedure

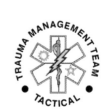

APPROVED
DATE: 01 OCT 06
Dr Kotwal
Dr Redman
Dr Cunningham
Dr Miles

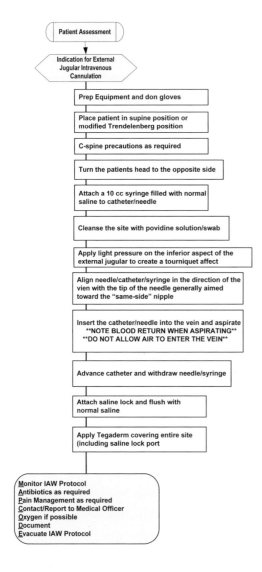

Patient Assessment

Indication for External Jugular Intravenous Cannulation

Prep Equipment and don gloves

Place patient in supine position or modified Trendelenberg position

C-spine precautions as required

Turn the patients head to the opposite side

Attach a 10 cc syringe filled with normal saline to catheter/needle

Cleanse the site with povidine solution/swab

Apply light pressure on the inferior aspect of the external jugular to create a tourniquet affect

Align needle/catheter/syringe in the direction of the vien with the tip of the needle generally aimed toward the "same-side" nipple

Insert the catheter/needle into the vein and aspirate
NOTE BLOOD RETURN WHEN ASPIRATING
DO NOT ALLOW AIR TO ENTER THE VEIN

Advance catheter and withdraw needle/syringe

Attach saline lock and flush with normal saline

Apply Tegaderm covering entire site (including saline lock port

Monitor IAW Protocol
Antibiotics as required
Pain Management as required
Contact/Report to Medical Officer
Oxygen if possible
Document
Evacuate IAW Protocol

EQUIPMENT NEEDED:
- Constricting Band
- Povidine-Iodine Swab
- 2 X 18-G IV Catheter/Needle
- 10 cc Syringe
- Saline Lock
- Tegaderm (at least 2.5" X 2.5")
- IV Tubing (10gtts/ml)
- Raptor/Linebacker securing device
- Tape, 2"
- Appropriate IV Fluids
- Gloves

DOCUMENTATION:
- ABC's
- Detailed Assessment
- Vital Signs
- SpO2
- IV Site
- IV Gauge
- Date/Time Started
- Fluids Infused / rate
- Complications Encountered

Sternal Intraosseous Infusion Procedure

Patient Assessment

↓

Indication for Sternal Intraosseous Infusion → Inability to attain vascular access through peripheral extremity or external jugular when life-saving fluids or medications are needed

Prep Equipment

Site Selection:
Adult Manubrium – Midline on the manubrium, 1.5 cm below the sternal notch

Prepare site with local anesthetic if PT is conscious

Cleanse site with povidine solution/swab

Use index finger of non-dominant hand to align the target patch with the patient's sternal notch

Verify Target Zone is on the midline over the manubrium Apply Patch

With patch securely attached to the patient's skin, the bone probe cluster is placed in the target zone, perpendicular to the skin

FAST-1 Insertion

With the introducer in hand, apply steady even pressure until infusion tube has penetrated the manubrium (release is felt)

Attach the infusion tube to the right angle female adapter and secure with protector dome

Attach syringe to the IV insertion site and aspirate bone marrow

Marrow Aspirates Freely? — NO → Flush the needle with 5 cc Normal Saline — Flushes Easily? — NO → Discontinue Procedure and find an alternate means of vascular access

YES ↓   YES ↓

Attach IV Tubing and/or saline lock

Secure Inducer Removal Package to the IV Line and/or Patient

Push needles of inducer into the accompanying sharps plug

Administer IV Fluids and/or Medications IAW appropriate protocol

Monitor IAW Protocol
Antibiotics as required
Pain Management as required
Contact/Report to Medical Officer
Oxygen if possible
Document
Evacuate IAW Protocol

EQUIPMENT NEEDED:
- FAST-1 Sternal Intraosseous (Complete)
  (6515-01-453-0960)

DOCUMENTATION:
- ABC's
- Detailed Assessment
- Vital Signs
- SpO2
- Complications Encountered

APPROVED
DATE: 01 OCT 06
Dr Kotwal
Dr Redman
Dr Cunningham
Dr Miles

Hypothermia Prevention & Management Kit Procedure

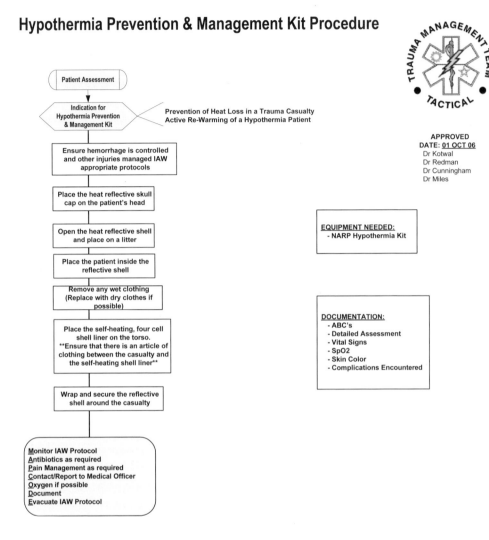

Patient Assessment

↓

Indication for Hypothermia Prevention & Management Kit

Prevention of Heat Loss in a Trauma Casualty
Active Re-Warming of a Hypothermia Patient

APPROVED
DATE: <u>01 OCT 06</u>
Dr Kotwal
Dr Redman
Dr Cunningham
Dr Miles

Ensure hemorrhage is controlled and other injuries managed IAW appropriate protocols

Place the heat reflective skull cap on the patient's head

Open the heat reflective shell and place on a litter

EQUIPMENT NEEDED:
- NARP Hypothermia Kit

Place the patient inside the reflective shell

Remove any wet clothing (Replace with dry clothes if possible)

Place the self-heating, four cell shell liner on the torso.
Ensure that there is an article of clothing between the casualty and the self-heating shell liner

DOCUMENTATION:
- ABC's
- Detailed Assessment
- Vital Signs
- SpO2
- Skin Color
- Complications Encountered

Wrap and secure the reflective shell around the casualty

<u>M</u>onitor IAW Protocol
<u>A</u>ntibiotics as required
<u>P</u>ain Management as required
<u>C</u>ontact/Report to Medical Officer
<u>O</u>xygen if possible
<u>D</u>ocument
<u>E</u>vacuate IAW Protocol

Head Injury Management Protocol

APPROVED
DATE: <u>01 OCT 06</u>
Dr Kotwal
Dr Redman
Dr Cunningham
Dr Miles

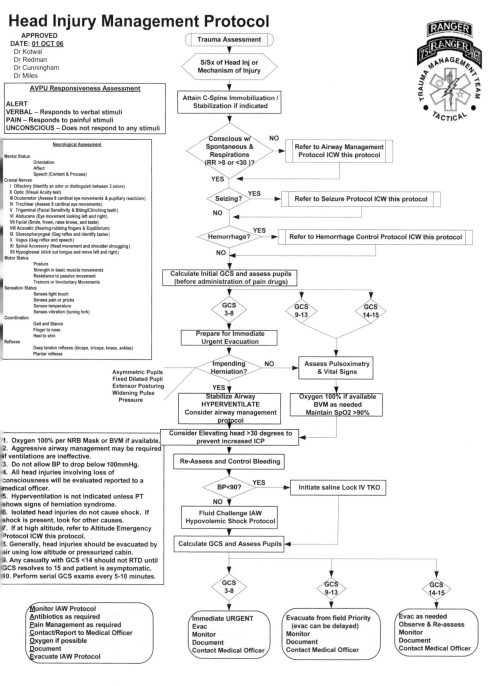

AVPU Responsiveness Assessment

ALERT
VERBAL – Responds to verbal stimuli
PAIN – Responds to painful stimuli
UNCONSCIOUS – Does not respond to any stimuli

Neurological Assessment

Mental Status
    Orientation
    Affect
    Speech (Content & Process)
Cranial Nerves
  I Olfactory (Identify an odor or distinguish between 2 odors)
  II Optic (Visual Acuity test)
  III Oculomotor (Assess 6 cardinal eye movements & pupillary reactcion)
  IV Trochlear (Assess 6 cardinal eye movements)
  V Trigeminal (Facial Sensitivity & Biting/Clinching teeth)
  VI Abducens (Eye movement looking left and right)
  VII Facial (Smile, frown, raise brows, and taste)
  VIII Acoustic (Hearing-rubbing fingers & Equilibrium)
  IX Glossopharyngeal (Gag reflex and identify tastes)
  X Vagus (Gag reflex and speech)
  XI Spinal Accessory (Head movement and shoulder shrugging)
  XII Hypoglossal (stick out tongue and move left and right)
Motor Status
    Posture
    Strength in basic muscle movements
    Resistance to passive movement
    Tremors or Involuntary Movements
Sensation Status
    Senses light touch
    Senses pain or pricks
    Senses temperature
    Senses vibration (tuning fork)
Coordination
    Gait and Stance
    Finger to nose
    Heel to shin
Reflexes
    Deep tendon reflexes (biceps, triceps, knees, ankles)
    Plantar reflexes

Trauma Assessment

S/Sx of Head Inj or Mechanism of Injury

Attain C-Spine Immobilization / Stabilization if indicated

Conscious w/ Spontaneous & Respirations (RR >8 or <30)? — NO → **Refer to Airway Management Protocol ICW this protocol**

YES

Seizing? — YES → **Refer to Seizure Protocol ICW this protocol**

NO

Hemorrhage? — YES → **Refer to Hemorrhage Control Protocol ICW this protocol**

NO

Calculate Initial GCS and assess pupils (before administration of pain drugs)

GCS 3-8   GCS 9-13   GCS 14-15

Prepare for Immediate Urgent Evacuation

Asymmetric Pupils
Fixed Dilated Pupil
Extensor Posturing
Widening Pulse Pressure

Impending Herniation? — NO → **Assess Pulsoximetry & Vital Signs**

YES

Stabilize Airway HYPERVENTILATE Consider airway management protocol

Oxygen 100% if available BVM as needed Maintain SpO2 >90%

1. Oxygen 100% per NRB Mask or BVM if available.
2. Aggressive airway management may be required if ventilations are ineffective.
3. Do not allow BP to drop below 100mmHg.
4. All head injuries involving loss of consciousness will be evaluated reported to a medical officer.
5. Hyperventilation is not indicated unless PT shows signs of herniation syndrome.
6. Isolated head injuries do not cause shock. If shock is present, look for other causes.
7. If at high altitude, refer to Altitude Emergency Protocol ICW this protocol.
8. Generally, head injuries should be evacuated by air using low altitude or pressurized cabin.
9. Any casualty with GCS <14 should not RTD until GCS resolves to 15 and patient is asymptomatic.
10. Perform serial GCS exams every 5-10 minutes.

Consider Elevating head >30 degrees to prevent increased ICP

Re-Assess and Control Bleeding

BP<90? — YES → **Initiate saline Lock IV TKO**

NO

Fluid Challenge IAW Hypovolemic Shock Protocol

Calculate GCS and Assess Pupils

GCS 3-8   GCS 9-13   GCS 14-15

Monitor IAW Protocol
Antibiotics as required
Pain Management as required
Contact/Report to Medical Officer
Oxygen if possible
Document
Evacuate IAW Protocol

Immediate URGENT Evac
Monitor
Document
Contact Medical Officer

Evacuate from field Priority (evac can be delayed)
Monitor
Document
Contact Medical Officer

Evac as needed
Observe & Re-assess
Monitor
Document
Contact Medical Officer

Mild Traumatic Brain Injury (Concussion) Management Protocol

Trauma Assessment

Post-Blast Screening of Involved Personnel

AVPU Responsiveness Assessment
ALERT
VERBAL – Responds to verbal stimuli
PAIN – Responds to painful stimuli
UNCONSCIOUS – Does not respond to any stimuli

S/Sx of mTBI or Mechanism of Injury

TBI Screening:
All personnel exposed to or involved in a blast, fall, vehicle crash or direct head impact who becomes dazed, confused or loses consciousness (even momentarily) should be further evaluated for brain injury.

Military Acute Concussion Evaluation (MACE)

I. Description of Incident. Ask:
  a. What happened?
  b. Tell me what you remember.
  c. Were you dazed or confused? Y or N
  d. Did you hit your head? Y or N

II. Cause of Injury. (All that apply)
  1. Explosion/Blast   5. Fall
  2. Blunt object   6. Gunshot wound
  3. Motor Vehicle Crash 7. Other_____
  4. Fragment

III. Was helmet worn? Y or N Type_____

IV. Amnesia Before: Are there any events just BEFORE the injury that are not remembered? Y or N How long?

V. Amnesia After: Are there any events just AFTER the injury that are not remembered? Y or N How long?

VI. Does the individual report loss of consciousness or "blacking out"? Y or N If yes, how long?_____

VII. Did anyone observe a period of loss of consciousness or unresponsiveness? Y or N If yes, how long? _____

VIII. Symptoms (All that apply)
  1. Headache   2. Dizziness
  3. Memory Problems   4. Balance problems
  5. Nausea/Vomiting   6. Difficulty Concentrating
  7. Irritability   8. Visual Disturbances
  9. Ringing in the ears 10. Other_____

EXAMINATION. Evaluate each domain. Total possible score is 30.
IX. Orientation (1 point each correct)
  Month   0   1
  Date   0   1
  Day of Week 0   1
  Year   0   1
  Time   0   1
          Orientation Total Score _____ of 5

X. Immediate Memory. Read all 5 words and ask PT to recall them in order. Repeat 2 more time times for a total of 3 trials. Score 1 point for each correct, over 3 trials.

LIST	Trial 1	Trial 2	Trial 3
Elbow	0 1	0 1	0 1
Apple	0 1	0 1	0 1
Carpet	0 1	0 1	0 1
Saddle	0 1	0 1	0 1
Bubble	0 1	0 1	0 1
Trial Score			

          Immediate Memory Total Score _____ of 15

XI. Neurological Screening. As the tactical & clinical situation permits, check:
  Eyes – pupillary response and tracking
  Verbal – speech fluency and word finding
  Motor – pronator drift, gait/coordination
  Record any abnormalities. No points for this section.

XII. Concentration. Reverse digits (go to next string length if correct on first trial. Stop if incorrect on both trials). 1 point for each correct string.
  4-9-3   0   1   6-2-9   0   1
  3-8-1-4   0   1   3-2-7-9   0   1
  6-2-9-7-1   0   1   1-5-2-8-5   0   1
  7-1-8-4-6-2 0   1   5-3-9-1-4-8   0   1

  Months in reverse order (1 point for entire sequence correct)
  Dec-Nov-Oct-Sep-Aug-Jul-Jun-May-Apr-Mar-Feb-Jan   0   1
          Concentration Total Score _____ of 5

XIII. Delayed Recall (1 point each) Ask the PT to recall the 5 words from the earlier memory test (DO NOT re-read the word list).
  Elbow   0   1
  Apple   0   1
  Carpet   0   1
  Saddle   0   1
  Bubble   0   1
          Delayed Recall Total Score _____ of 5

TOTAL SCORE _____ of 30

Attain C-Spine Immobilization / Stabilization if indicated and possible

Obvious Life Threatening Injuries? — YES → **DEFER to appropriate trauma protocols**

NO ↓

S/Sx or Suspected Concussion? — NO → Educate individual or group on concussion syndrome with instructions to return for care if displaying signs and symptoms. If a patient returns, then start protocol from beginning.

YES ↓

Report to medical officer if possible

Evaluate for Red Flag Indicators and MACE (Parts IV-VIII)

RED FLAG SIGNS & SYMPTOMS
Worsening mental status
Pupillary asymetry
Seizures
Repeated vomiting
Double vision   Worsening headache
Unusual behavior   Disoriented to person/place
Confused or irritable   Slurred speech
Unsteady on feet   Weakness/numbness to
extremities

Red Flag Indicators Present or PT has had a recent concussion? — YES →

NO ↓

Tylenol PRN No narcotics/analgesics unless indicated by other injuries

Administer Full MACE

MACE <25 or positive findings on parts IV-VIII? — YES → **Evacuate to Higher Medical Capability**

NO ↓

Exertional exercise testing for 5 minutes (PU/SU/Run-in-place)

Determine Evacuation Precedence

MACE <25 or positive symptoms on part VIII? — YES →

NO ↓

URGENT
Declining Level of Consciousness or Mental Status
Pupillary Asymmetry
Seizures
Breathing Difficulties

PRIORITY
Double Vision
Worsening Headache
Disorientation to Person/Place/Time
Unusual Behavior
Confusion or Irritable
Slurred Speech
Unsteady on feet or gait
Repeated vomiting
Weakness or Numbness to extremities

Repeat testing every 12-24 hours. RTD after at least 24 hours post-injury and PT has met RTD criteria

Return To Duty Criteria:
No Signs & Symptoms
MACE Negative (score >25)
Resting Signs & Symptoms Negative
Exertion Signs & Symptoms Negative

Monitor IAW Protocol
Antibiotics as required
Pain Management as required
Contact/Report to Medical Officer
Oxygen if possible
Document
Evacuate IAW Protocol

Evacuate as needed or directed

2-20

Seizure Management Protocol

APPROVED
DATE: 01 OCT 06
Dr Kotwal
Dr Redman
Dr Cunningham
Dr Miles

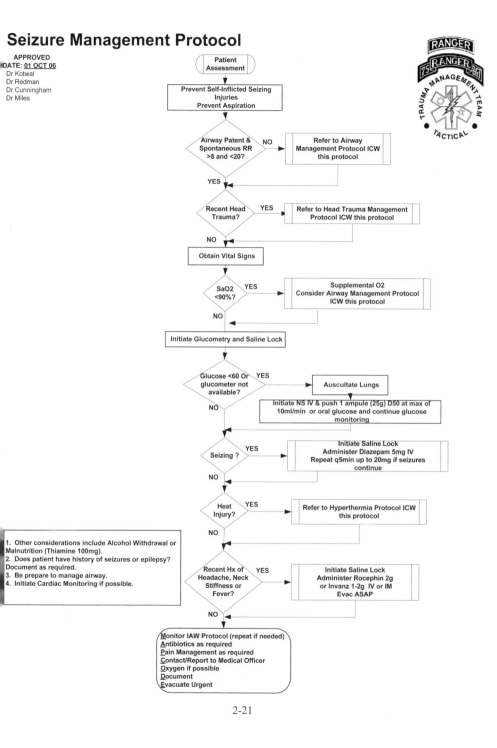

1. Other considerations include Alcohol Withdrawal or Malnutrition (Thiamine 100mg).
2. Does patient have history of seizures or epilepsy? Document as required.
3. Be prepare to manage airway.
4. Initiate Cardiac Monitoring if possible.

Patient Assessment

Prevent Self-Inflicted Seizing Injuries
Prevent Aspiration

Airway Patent & Spontaneous RR >8 and <20? — NO → Refer to Airway Management Protocol ICW this protocol

YES

Recent Head Trauma? — YES → Refer to Head Trauma Management Protocol ICW this protocol

NO

Obtain Vital Signs

SaO2 <90%? — YES → Supplemental O2 Consider Airway Management Protocol ICW this protocol

NO

Initiate Glucometry and Saline Lock

Glucose <60 Or glucometer not available? — YES → Auscultate Lungs

Initiate NS IV & push 1 ampule (25g) D50 at max of 10ml/min or oral glucose and continue glucose monitoring

NO

Seizing ? — YES → Initiate Saline Lock
Administer Diazepam 5mg IV
Repeat q5min up to 20mg if seizures continue

NO

Heat Injury? — YES → Refer to Hyperthermia Protocol ICW this protocol

NO

Recent Hx of Headache, Neck Stiffness or Fever? — YES → Initiate Saline Lock
Administer Rocephin 2g or Invanz 1-2g IV or IM
Evac ASAP

NO

Monitor IAW Protocol (repeat if needed)
Antibiotics as required
Pain Management as required
Contact/Report to Medical Officer
Oxygen if possible
Document
Evacuate Urgent

Spinal Cord Injury Management Protocol

APPROVED
DATE: 01 OCT 06
Dr Kotwal
Dr Redman
Dr Cunningham
Dr Miles

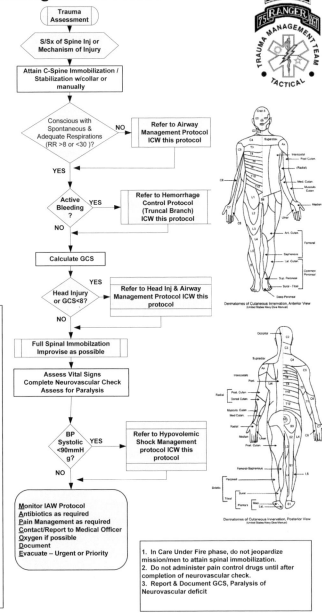

AVPU Responsiveness Assessment

ALERT
VERBAL – Responds to verbal stimuli
PAIN – Responds to painful stimuli
UNCONSCIOUS – Does not respond to any stimuli

Glasgow Coma Scale

Eye Opening	Spontaneous	4
	To Voice	3
	To Pain	2
	None	1
Verbal Response	Oriented	5
	Confused	4
	Inappropriate Words	3
	Incomprehensible Words	2
	None	1
Motor Response	Obeys Commands	6
	Localizes Pain	5
	Withdraws (Pain)	4
	Flexion	3
	Extension	2
	None	1

Document as: E___ + V___ + M___ = ___

Neurological Assessment

Mental Status
    Orientation
    Affect
    Speech (Content & Process)
Cranial Nerves
  I Olfactory (Identify an odor or distinguish between 2 odors)
  II Optic (Visual Acuity test)
  III Oculomotor (Assess 6 cardinal eye movements & pupillary reactcion)
  IV Trochlear (Assess 6 cardinal eye movements)
  V Trigeminal (Facial Sensitivity & Biting/Clinching teeth)
  VI Abducens (Eye movement looking left and right)
  VII Facial (Smile, frown, raise brows, and taste)
  VIII Vestibulocochlear (Hearing-rubbing fingers & Equilibrium)
  IX Acoustic (Gag reflex and identify tastes)
  X Vagus (Gag reflex and speech)
  XI Spinal Accessory (Head movement and shoulder shrugging)
  XII Hypoglossal (stick out tongue and move left and right)
Motor Status
    Posture
    Strength in basic muscle movements
    Resistance to passive movement
    Tremors or Involuntary Movements
Sensation Status
    Senses light touch
    Senses pain or pricks
    Senses temperature
    Senses vibration (tuning fork)
Coordination
    Gait and Stance
    Finger to nose
    Heel to shin
Reflexes
    Deep tendon reflexes (biceps, triceps, knees, ankles)
    Plantar reflexes

Trauma Assessment

S/Sx of Spine Inj or Mechanism of Injury

Attain C-Spine Immobilization / Stabilization w/collar or manually

Conscious with Spontaneous & Adequate Respirations (RR >8 or <30)? — NO → **Refer to Airway Management Protocol ICW this protocol**

YES

Active Bleeding ? — YES → **Refer to Hemorrhage Control Protocol (Truncal Branch) ICW this protocol**

NO

Calculate GCS

Head Injury or GCS<8? — YES → **Refer to Head Inj & Airway Management Protocol ICW this protocol**

NO

Full Spinal Immobilzation Improvise as possible

Assess Vital Signs Complete Neurovascular Check Assess for Paralysis

BP Systolic <90mmHg? — YES → **Refer to Hypovolemic Shock Management protocol ICW this protocol**

NO

U**nderline**: **Monitor IAW Protocol**
Antibiotics as required
Pain Management as required
Contact/Report to Medical Officer
Oxygen if possible
Document
Evacuate – Urgent or Priority

1. In Care Under Fire phase, do not jeopardize mission/men to attain spinal immobilization.
2. Do not administer pain control drugs until after completion of neurovascular check.
3. Report & Document GCS, Paralysis of Neurovascular deficit

Dermatomes of Cutaneous Innervation, Anterior View
(United States Navy Dive Manual)

Dermatomes of Cutaneous Innervation, Posterior View
(United States Navy Dive Manual)

Orthopedic Trauma Management Protocol

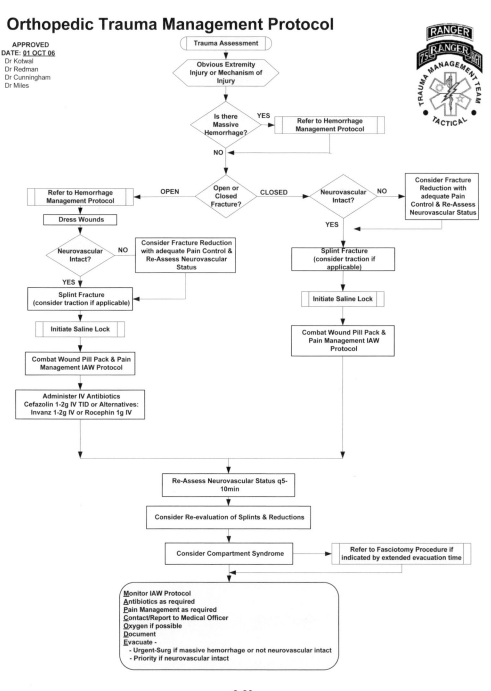

APPROVED
DATE: <u>01 OCT 06</u>
Dr Kotwal
Dr Redman
Dr Cunningham
Dr Miles

Trauma Assessment

Obvious Extremity Injury or Mechanism of Injury

Is there Massive Hemorrhage? — YES → Refer to Hemorrhage Management Protocol

NO

Open or Closed Fracture?

OPEN → Refer to Hemorrhage Management Protocol → Dress Wounds

Neurovascular Intact? — NO → Consider Fracture Reduction with adequate Pain Control & Re-Assess Neurovascular Status

YES → Splint Fracture (consider traction if applicable) → Initiate Saline Lock → Combat Wound Pill Pack & Pain Management IAW Protocol → Administer IV Antibiotics Cefazolin 1-2g IV TID or Alternatives: Invanz 1-2g IV or Rocephin 1g IV

CLOSED → Neurovascular Intact? — NO → Consider Fracture Reduction with adequate Pain Control & Re-Assess Neurovascular Status

YES → Splint Fracture (consider traction if applicable) → Initiate Saline Lock → Combat Wound Pill Pack & Pain Management IAW Protocol

Re-Assess Neurovascular Status q5-10min

Consider Re-evaluation of Splints & Reductions

Consider Compartment Syndrome → Refer to Fasciotomy Procedure if indicated by extended evacuation time

Monitor IAW Protocol
Antibiotics as required
Pain Management as required
Contact/Report to Medical Officer
Oxygen if possible
Document
Evacuate -
  - Urgent-Surg if massive hemorrhage or not neurovascular intact
  - Priority if neurovascular intact

2-23

Burn Management Protocol

APPROVED
DATE: 01 OCT 06
Dr Kotwal
Dr Redman
Dr Cunningham
Dr Miles

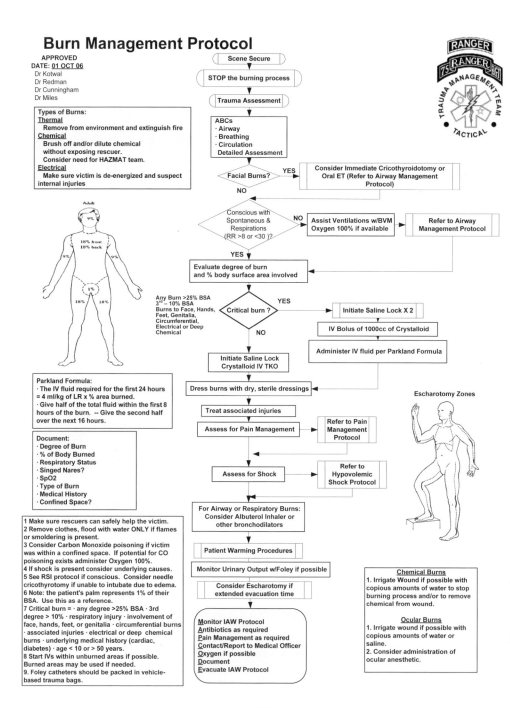

Types of Burns:
Thermal
  Remove from environment and extinguish fire
Chemical
  Brush off and/or dilute chemical without exposing rescuer.
  Consider need for HAZMAT team.
Electrical
  Make sure victim is de-energized and suspect internal injuries

Scene Secure

STOP the burning process

Trauma Assessment

ABCs
· Airway
· Breathing
· Circulation
Detailed Assessment

Facial Burns? — YES → Consider Immediate Cricothyroidotomy or Oral ET (Refer to Airway Management Protocol)

NO

Conscious with Spontaneous & Respirations (RR >8 or <30)? — NO → Assist Ventilations w/BVM Oxygen 100% if available → Refer to Airway Management Protocol

YES

Evaluate degree of burn and % body surface area involved

Any Burn >25% BSA
3rd – 10% BSA
Burns to Face, Hands, Feet, Genitalia, Circumferential, Electrical or Deep Chemical

Critical burn ? — YES → Initiate Saline Lock X 2

IV Bolus of 1000cc of Crystalloid

Administer IV fluid per Parkland Formula

NO

Initiate Saline Lock Crystalloid IV TKO

Dress burns with dry, sterile dressings

Parkland Formula:
· The IV fluid required for the first 24 hours = 4 ml/kg of LR x % area burned.
· Give half of the total fluid within the first 8 hours of the burn. -- Give the second half over the next 16 hours.

Treat associated injuries

Assess for Pain Management → Refer to Pain Management Protocol

Document:
· Degree of Burn
· % of Body Burned
· Respiratory Status
· Singed Nares?
· SpO2
· Type of Burn
· Medical History
· Confined Space?

Assess for Shock → Refer to Hypovolemic Shock Protocol

For Airway or Respiratory Burns: Consider Albuterol Inhaler or other bronchodilators

Patient Warming Procedures

Monitor Urinary Output w/Foley if possible

Consider Escharotomy if extended evacuation time

1 Make sure rescuers can safely help the victim.
2 Remove clothes, flood with water ONLY if flames or smoldering is present.
3 Consider Carbon Monoxide poisoning if victim was within a confined space. If potential for CO poisoning exists administer Oxygen 100%.
4 If shock is present consider underlying causes.
5 See RSI protocol if conscious. Consider needle cricothyrotomy if unable to intubate due to edema.
6 Note: the patient's palm represents 1% of their BSA. Use this as a reference.
7 Critical burn = · any degree >25% BSA · 3rd degree > 10% · respiratory injury · involvement of face, hands, feet, or genitalia · circumferential burns · associated injuries · electrical or deep chemical burns · underlying medical history (cardiac, diabetes) · age < 10 or > 50 years.
8 Start IVs within unburned areas if possible. Burned areas may be used if needed.
9. Foley catheters should be packed in vehicle-based trauma bags.

Monitor IAW Protocol
Antibiotics as required
Pain Management as required
Contact/Report to Medical Officer
Oxygen if possible
Document
Evacuate IAW Protocol

Escharotomy Zones

Chemical Burns
1. Irrigate Wound if possible with copious amounts of water to stop burning process and/or to remove chemical from wound.

Ocular Burns
1. Irrigate wound if possible with copious amounts of water or saline.
2. Consider administration of ocular anesthetic.

Foley Catheterization Procedure

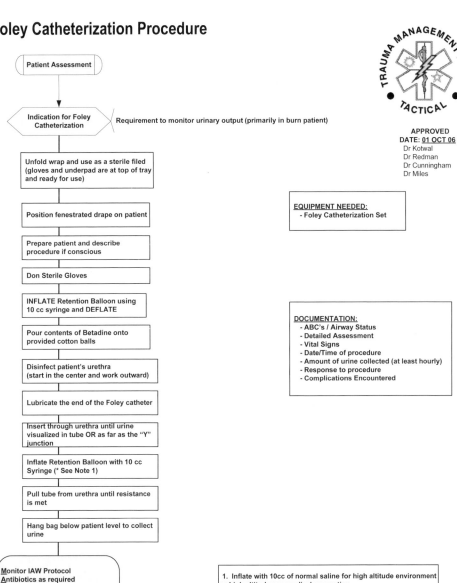

Patient Assessment

Indication for Foley Catheterization — Requirement to monitor urinary output (primarily in burn patient)

Unfold wrap and use as a sterile filed (gloves and underpad are at top of tray and ready for use)

Position fenestrated drape on patient

Prepare patient and describe procedure if conscious

Don Sterile Gloves

INFLATE Retention Balloon using 10 cc syringe and DEFLATE

Pour contents of Betadine onto provided cotton balls

Disinfect patient's urethra (start in the center and work outward)

Lubricate the end of the Foley catheter

Insert through urethra until urine visualized in tube OR as far as the "Y" junction

Inflate Retention Balloon with 10 cc Syringe (* See Note 1)

Pull tube from urethra until resistance is met

Hang bag below patient level to collect urine

Monitor IAW Protocol
Antibiotics as required
Pain Management as required
Contact/Report to Medical Officer
Oxygen if possible
Document
Evacuate IAW Protocol

TRAUMA MANAGEMENT TEAM TACTICAL

APPROVED
DATE: 01 OCT 06
Dr Kotwal
Dr Redman
Dr Cunningham
Dr Miles

EQUIPMENT NEEDED:
- Foley Catheterization Set

DOCUMENTATION:
- ABC's / Airway Status
- Detailed Assessment
- Vital Signs
- Date/Time of procedure
- Amount of urine collected (at least hourly)
- Response to procedure
- Complications Encountered

1. Inflate with 10cc of normal saline for high altitude environment or high altitude aeromedical evacuation.

Pain Management Protocol

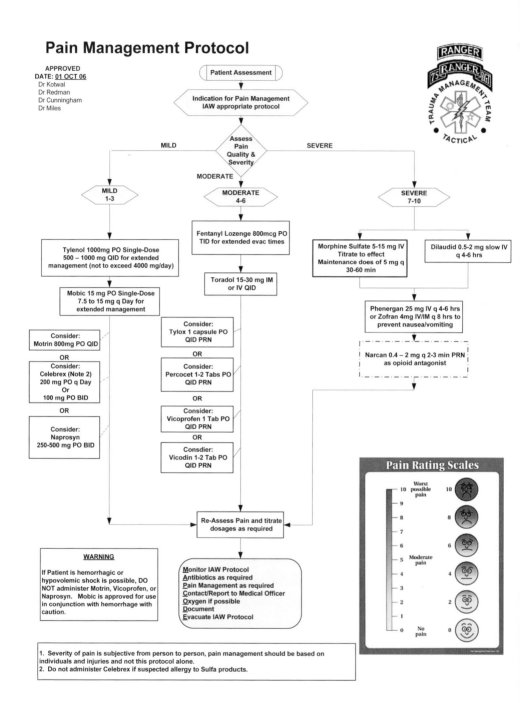

APPROVED
DATE: 01 OCT 06
Dr Kotwal
Dr Redman
Dr Cunningham
Dr Miles

Patient Assessment

Indication for Pain Management IAW appropriate protocol

Assess Pain Quality & Severity

MILD — MODERATE — SEVERE

MILD 1-3

MODERATE 4-6

SEVERE 7-10

Tylenol 1000mg PO Single-Dose 500 – 1000 mg QID for extended management (not to exceed 4000 mg/day)

Fentanyl Lozenge 800mcg PO TID for extended evac times

Morphine Sulfate 5-15 mg IV Titrate to effect Maintenance does of 5 mg q 30-60 min

Dilaudid 0.5-2 mg slow IV q 4-6 hrs

Mobic 15 mg PO Single-Dose 7.5 to 15 mg q Day for extended management

Toradol 15-30 mg IM or IV QID

Phenergan 25 mg IV q 4-6 hrs or Zofran 4mg IV/IM q 8 hrs to prevent nausea/vomiting

Consider: Motrin 800mg PO QID

OR

Consider: Celebrex (Note 2) 200 mg PO q Day Or 100 mg PO BID

OR

Consider: Naprosyn 250-500 mg PO BID

Consider: Tylox 1 capsule PO QID PRN

OR

Consider: Percocet 1-2 Tabs PO QID PRN

OR

Consider: Vicoprofen 1 Tab PO QID PRN

OR

Consdier: Vicodin 1-2 Tab PO QID PRN

Narcan 0.4 – 2 mg q 2-3 min PRN as opioid antagonist

Re-Assess Pain and titrate dosages as required

WARNING

If Patient is hemorrhagic or hypovolemic shock is possible, DO NOT administer Motrin, Vicoprofen, or Naprosyn. Mobic is approved for use in conjunction with hemorrhage with caution.

Monitor IAW Protocol
Antibiotics as required
Pain Management as required
Contact/Report to Medical Officer
Oxygen if possible
Document
Evacuate IAW Protocol

Pain Rating Scales

10 Worst possible pain	10
9	
8	8
7	
6	6
5 Moderate pain	
4	4
3	
2	2
1	
0 No pain	0

1. Severity of pain is subjective from person to person, pain management should be based on individuals and injuries and not this protocol alone.
2. Do not administer Celebrex if suspected allergy to Sulfa products.

Anaphylactic Shock Management Protocol

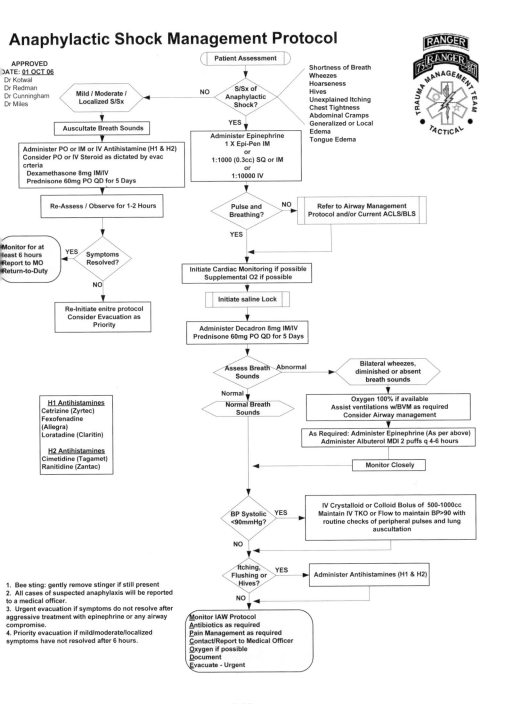

APPROVED
DATE: 01 OCT 06
Dr Kotwal
Dr Redman
Dr Cunningham
Dr Miles

Patient Assessment

S/Sx of Anaphylactic Shock?

Shortness of Breath
Wheezes
Hoarseness
Hives
Unexplained Itching
Chest Tightness
Abdominal Cramps
Generalized or Local Edema
Tongue Edema

NO → Mild / Moderate / Localized S/Sx

Auscultate Breath Sounds

Administer PO or IM or IV Antihistamine (H1 & H2)
Consider PO or IV Steroid as dictated by evac crteria
   Dexamethasone 8mg IM/IV
   Prednisone 60mg PO QD for 5 Days

Re-Assess / Observe for 1-2 Hours

Symptoms Resolved?
YES → Monitor for at least 6 hours
Report to MO
Return-to-Duty

NO → Re-Initiate enitre protocol
Consider Evacuation as Priority

YES → Administer Epinephrine
1 X Epi-Pen IM
or
1:1000 (0.3cc) SQ or IM
or
1:10000 IV

Pulse and Breathing?
NO → Refer to Airway Management Protocol and/or Current ACLS/BLS

YES

Initiate Cardiac Monitoring if possible
Supplemental O2 if possible

Initiate saline Lock

Administer Decadron 8mg IM/IV
Prednisone 60mg PO QD for 5 Days

Assess Breath Sounds
Abnormal → Bilateral wheezes, diminished or absent breath sounds

Normal → Normal Breath Sounds

Oxygen 100% if available
Assist ventilations w/BVM as required
Consider Airway management

As Required: Administer Epinephrine (As per above)
Administer Albuterol MDI 2 puffs q 4-6 hours

Monitor Closely

H1 Antihistamines
Cetrizine (Zyrtec)
Fexofenadine (Allegra)
Loratadine (Claritin)

H2 Antihistamines
Cimetidine (Tagamet)
Ranitidine (Zantac)

BP Systolic <90mmHg?
YES → IV Crystalloid or Colloid Bolus of 500-1000cc
Maintain IV TKO or Flow to maintain BP>90 with routine checks of peripheral pulses and lung auscultation

NO

Itching, Flushing or Hives?
YES → Administer Antihistamines (H1 & H2)

NO

Monitor IAW Protocol
Antibiotics as required
Pain Management as required
Contact/Report to Medical Officer
Oxygen if possible
Document
Evacuate - Urgent

1. Bee sting: gently remove stinger if still present
2. All cases of suspected anaphylaxis will be reported to a medical officer.
3. Urgent evacuation if symptoms do not resolve after aggressive treatment with epinephrine or any airway compromise.
4. Priority evacuation if mild/moderate/localized symptoms have not resolved after 6 hours.

Hyperthermia (Heat) Management Protocol

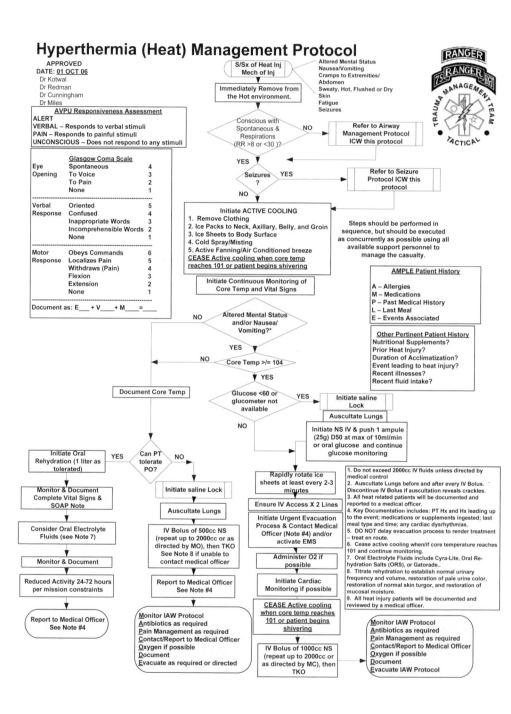

APPROVED
DATE: 01 OCT 06
Dr Kotwal
Dr Redman
Dr Cunningham
Dr Miles

AVPU Responsiveness Assessment
ALERT
VERBAL – Responds to verbal stimuli
PAIN – Responds to painful stimuli
UNCONSCIOUS – Does not respond to any stimuli

Glasgow Coma Scale

Eye Opening	Spontaneous	4
	To Voice	3
	To Pain	2
	None	1
Verbal Response	Oriented	5
	Confused	4
	Inappropriate Words	3
	Incomprehensible Words	2
	None	1
Motor Response	Obeys Commands	6
	Localizes Pain	5
	Withdraws (Pain)	4
	Flexion	3
	Extension	2
	None	1

Document as: E___ + V___ + M___ = ___

S/Sx of Heat Inj Mech of Inj
Altered Mental Status
Nausea/Vomiting
Cramps to Extremities/ Abdomen
Sweaty, Hot, Flushed or Dry Skin
Fatigue
Seizures

Immediately Remove from the Hot environment.

Conscious with Spontaneous & Respirations (RR >8 or <30)? — NO → Refer to Airway Management Protocol ICW this protocol

YES

Seizures? — YES → Refer to Seizure Protocol ICW this protocol

NO

Initiate ACTIVE COOLING
1. Remove Clothing
2. Ice Packs to Neck, Axillary, Belly, and Groin
3. Ice Sheets to Body Surface
4. Cold Spray/Misting
5. Active Fanning/Air Conditioned breeze
CEASE Active cooling when core temp reaches 101 or patient begins shivering

Steps should be performed in sequence, but should be executed as concurrently as possible using all available support personnel to manage the casualty.

Initiate Continuous Monitoring of Core Temp and Vital Signs

AMPLE Patient History
A – Allergies
M – Medications
P – Past Medical History
L – Last Meal
E – Events Associated

Other Pertinent Patient History
Nutritional Supplements?
Prior Heat Injury?
Duration of Acclimatization?
Event leading to heat injury?
Recent illnesses?
Recent fluid intake?

Altered Mental Status and/or Nausea/ Vomiting?* — NO

YES

Core Temp >/= 104 — NO

YES

Document Core Temp

Glucose <60 or glucometer not available — YES → Initiate saline Lock

Auscultate Lungs

NO

Initiate NS IV & push 1 ampule (25g) D50 at max of 10ml/min or oral glucose and continue glucose monitoring

Can PT tolerate PO? — YES → Initiate Oral Rehydration (1 liter as tolerated)

NO

Monitor & Document Complete Vital Signs & SOAP Note

Consider Oral Electrolyte Fluids (see Note 7)

Monitor & Document

Reduced Activity 24-72 hours per mission constraints

Report to Medical Officer See Note #4

Initiate saline Lock

Auscultate Lungs

IV Bolus of 500cc NS (repeat up to 2000cc or as directed by MO), then TKO See Note 8 if unable to contact medical officer

Report to Medical Officer See Note #4

Monitor IAW Protocol
Antibiotics as required
Pain Management as required
Contact/Report to Medical Officer
Oxygen if possible
Document
Evacuate as required or directed

Rapidly rotate ice sheets at least every 2-3 minutes

Ensure IV Access X 2 Lines

Initiate Urgent Evacuation Process & Contact Medical Officer (Note #4) and/or activate EMS

Administer O2 if possible

Initiate Cardiac Monitoring if possible

CEASE Active cooling when core temp reaches 101 or patient begins shivering

IV Bolus of 1000cc NS (repeat up to 2000cc as directed by MC), then TKO

1. Do not exceed 2000cc IV fluids unless directed by medical control
2. Auscultate Lungs before and after every IV Bolus. Discontinue IV Bolus if auscultation reveals crackles.
3. All heat related patients will be documented and reported to a medical officer.
4. Key Documentation includes: PT Hx and Hx leading up to the event; medications or supplements ingested; last meal type and time; any cardiac dysrhythmias.
5. DO NOT delay evacuation process to render treatment – treat en route.
6. Cease active cooling when/if core temperature reaches 101 and continue monitoring.
7. Oral Electrolyte Fluids include Cyra-Lite, Oral Re-hydration Salts (ORS), or Gatorade..
8. Titrate rehydration to establish normal urinary frequency and volume, restoration of pale urine color, restoration of normal skin turgor, and restoration of mucosal moisture.
9. All heat injury patients will be documented and reviewed by a medical officer.

Monitor IAW Protocol
Antibiotics as required
Pain Management as required
Contact/Report to Medical Officer
Oxygen if possible
Document
Evacuate IAW Protocol

Hypothermia Prevention & Management Protocol

APPROVED
DATE: 01 OCT 06
Dr Kotwal
Dr Redman
Dr Cunningham
Dr Miles

Patient Assessment

↓

S/Sx of Hypothermia or
Cold Weather Injury

↓

Assess Responsiveness
Airway
Breathing
Circulation

↓

- Remove wet clothing
- Prevent heat loss/wind chill
- Maintain horizontal position
- Avoid rough movement
- Monitor core temperature
- Monitor cardiac rhythm

↓

Pulse &
Breathng
?

NO →

Start CPR
Refer to current ACLS Guidelines
Defibrillate if available
 - 1 X shock at 360J (monophasic) or 150J
   (biphasic)
Refer to Airway Management Protocol
Ventilate with warm, humid O2 if available
Repeat defibrillation if core temp >86
Continue CPR as required

YES

↓

Assess Core Temperature ←

↓

Active External Re-warming
-Blizzard Blanket
-Ranger Rescue Wrap
-Thermo-Lite
-Ranger Buddy/Sleeping Bag

↓

Consider Active Internal Re-warming
- Warm IV fluid
 - Thermal Angel
 - MRE Heater
- Warm, humidified oxygen if available

↓

- Notify receiving hospital ASAP
- Monitor Cardiac Rhythm,
  Core Temp, VS, SpO2
- Support Respiratory Effort
- Transport ASAP

↓

Monitor IAW Protocol
Antibiotics as required
Pain Management as required
Contact/Report to Medical Officer
Oxygen if possible
Document
Evacuate IAW Protocol

Document:
- Signs & Symptoms
- Vital Signs, SpO2
- Cardiac Rhythm
- Core Temp
- Mechanism of Injury
- Treatment
- Response to Treatment

1 Other Methods include: electrical or charcoal warming devices, hot
  water baths, heating pads, radiant heat sources and warming beds.
2 Give IV medications at longer than standard intervals.
3 Do not defibrillate a second time until core temperature >86F

Behavioral Emergency Management Protocol

APPROVED
DATE: 01 OCT 06
Dr Kotwal
Dr Redman
Dr Cunningham
Dr Miles

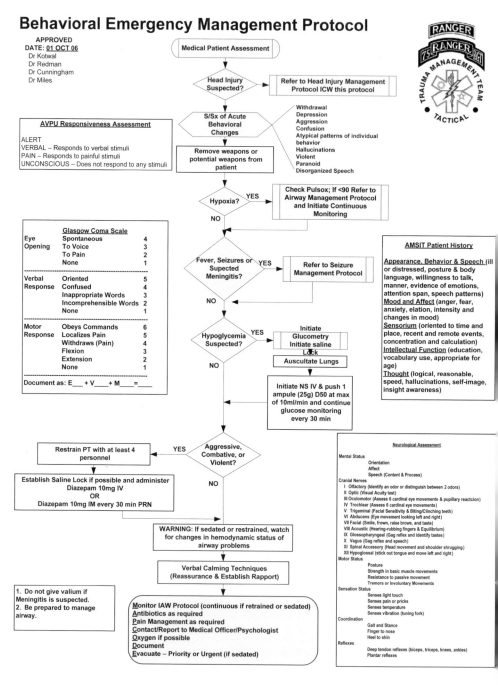

Medical Patient Assessment

Head Injury Suspected? → **Refer to Head Injury Management Protocol ICW this protocol**

S/Sx of Acute Behavioral Changes:
- Withdrawal
- Depression
- Aggression
- Confusion
- Atypical patterns of individual behavior
- Hallucinations
- Violent
- Paranoid
- Disorganized Speech

Remove weapons or potential weapons from patient

AVPU Responsiveness Assessment

ALERT
VERBAL – Responds to verbal stimuli
PAIN – Responds to painful stimuli
UNCONSCIOUS – Does not respond to any stimuli

Hypoxia? — YES → **Check Pulsox; If <90 Refer to Airway Management Protocol and Initiate Continuous Monitoring**

NO

Fever, Seizures or Suspected Meningitis? — YES → **Refer to Seizure Management Protocol**

NO

Glasgow Coma Scale		
Eye Opening	Spontaneous	4
	To Voice	3
	To Pain	2
	None	1
Verbal Response	Oriented	5
	Confused	4
	Inappropriate Words	3
	Incomprehensible Words	2
	None	1
Motor Response	Obeys Commands	6
	Localizes Pain	5
	Withdraws (Pain)	4
	Flexion	3
	Extension	2
	None	1

Document as: E___ + V___ + M___ = ___

Hypoglycemia Suspected? — YES → **Initiate Glucometry Initiate saline Lock**

Auscultate Lungs

NO

Initiate NS IV & push 1 ampule (25g) D50 at max of 10ml/min and continue glucose monitoring every 30 min

Aggressive, Combative, or Violent? — YES → **Restrain PT with at least 4 personnel**

Establish Saline Lock if possible and administer Diazepam 10mg IV OR Diazepam 10mg IM every 30 min PRN

NO

WARNING: If sedated or restrained, watch for changes in hemodynamic status of airway problems

Verbal Calming Techniques (Reassurance & Establish Rapport)

1. Do not give valium if Meningitis is suspected.
2. Be prepared to manage airway.

Monitor IAW Protocol (continuous if retrained or sedated)
Antibiotics as required
Pain Management as required
Contact/Report to Medical Officer/Psychologist
Oxygen if possible
Document
Evacuate – Priority or Urgent (if sedated)

AMSIT Patient History

Appearance, Behavior & Speech (ill or distressed, posture & body language, willingness to talk, manner, evidence of emotions, attention span, speech patterns)
Mood and Affect (anger, fear, anxiety, elation, intensity and changes in mood)
Sensorium (oriented to time and place, recent and remote events, concentration and calculation)
Intellectual Function (education, vocabulary use, appropriate for age)
Thought (logical, reasonable, speed, hallucinations, self-image, insight awareness)

Neurological Assessment

Mental Status
    Orientation
    Affect
    Speech (Content & Process)
Cranial Nerves
    I Olfactory (Identify an odor or distinguish between 2 odors)
    II Optic (Visual Acuity test)
    III Oculomotor (Assess 6 cardinal eye movements & pupillary reaction)
    IV Trochlear (Assess 6 cardinal eye movements)
    V Trigeminal (Facial Sensitivity & Biting/Clinching teeth)
    VI Abducens (Eye movement looking left and right)
    VII Facial (Smile, frown, raise brows, and taste)
    VIII Acoustic (Hearing-rubbing fingers & Equilibrium)
    IX Glossopharyngeal (Gag reflex and identify tastes)
    X Vagus (Gag reflex and speech)
    XI Spinal Accessory (Head movement and shoulder shrugging)
    XII Hypoglossal (stick out tongue and move left and right)
Motor Status
    Posture
    Strength in basic muscle movements
    Resistance to passive movement
    Tremors or Involuntary Movements
Sensation Status
    Senses light touch
    Senses pain or pricks
    Senses temperature
    Senses vibration (tuning fork)
Coordination
    Gait and Stance
    Finger to nose
    Heel to shin
Reflexes
    Deep tendon reflexes (biceps, triceps, knees, ankles)
    Plantar reflexes

Altitude Medical Emergency Management Protocol

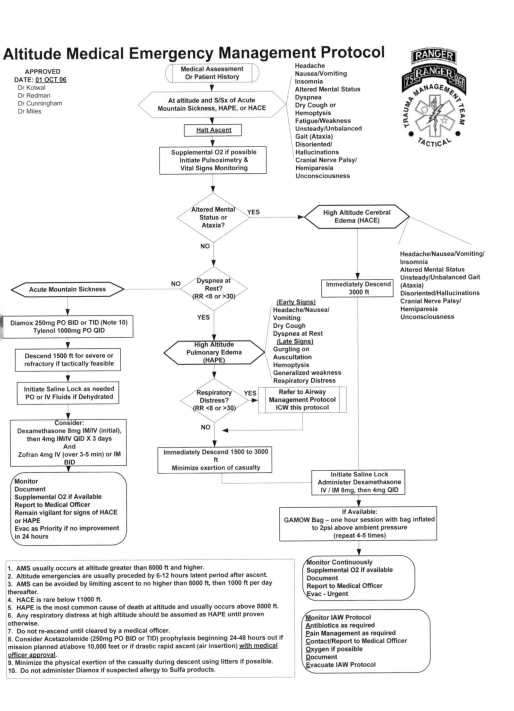

APPROVED
DATE: 01 OCT 06
Dr Kotwal
Dr Redman
Dr Cunningham
Dr Miles

Medical Assessment Or Patient History

At altitude and S/Sx of Acute Mountain Sickness, HAPE, or HACE

Headache
Nausea/Vomiting
Insomnia
Altered Mental Status
Dyspnea
Dry Cough or Hemoptysis
Fatigue/Weakness
Unsteady/Unbalanced Gait (Ataxia)
Disoriented/Hallucinations
Cranial Nerve Palsy/Hemiparesia
Unconsciousness

Halt Ascent

Supplemental O2 if possible
Initiate Pulsoximetry & Vital Signs Monitoring

Altered Mental Status or Ataxia? **YES** → High Altitude Cerebral Edema (HACE)

NO

Dyspnea at Rest? (RR <8 or >30) **NO** → Acute Mountain Sickness

Headache/Nausea/Vomiting/
Insomnia
Altered Mental Status
Unsteady/Unbalanced Gait (Ataxia)
Disoriented/Hallucinations
Cranial Nerve Palsy/Hemiparesia
Unconsciousness

Immediately Descend 3000 ft

Acute Mountain Sickness:
Diamox 250mg PO BID or TID (Note 10)
Tylenol 1000mg PO QID

Descend 1500 ft for severe or refractory if tactically feasible

Initiate Saline Lock as needed
PO or IV Fluids if Dehydrated

Consider:
Dexamethasone 8mg IM/IV (initial), then 4mg IM/IV QID X 3 days
And
Zofran 4mg IV (over 3-5 min) or IM BID

Monitor
Document
Supplemental O2 if Available
Report to Medical Officer
Remain vigilant for signs of HACE or HAPE
Evac as Priority if no improvement in 24 hours

YES

High Altitude Pulmonary Edema (HAPE)

(Early Signs)
Headache/Nausea/
Vomiting
Dry Cough
Dyspnea at Rest
(Late Signs)
Gurgling on Auscultation
Hemoptysis
Generalized weakness
Respiratory Distress

Respiratory Distress? (RR <8 or >30) **YES** → Refer to Airway Management Protocol ICW this protocol

NO

Immediately Descend 1500 to 3000 ft
Minimize exertion of casualty

Initiate Saline Lock
Administer Dexamethasone IV / IM 8mg, then 4mg QID

If Available:
GAMOW Bag – one hour session with bag inflated to 2psi above ambient pressure
(repeat 4-5 times)

Monitor Continuously
Supplemental O2 if available
Document
Report to Medical Officer
Evac - Urgent

Monitor IAW Protocol
Antibiotics as required
Pain Management as required
Contact/Report to Medical Officer
Oxygen if possible
Document
Evacuate IAW Protocol

1. AMS usually occurs at altitude greater than 8000 ft and higher.
2. Altitude emergencies are usually preceded by 6-12 hours latent period after ascent.
3. AMS can be avoided by limiting ascent to no higher than 8000 ft, then 1000 ft per day thereafter.
4. HACE is rare below 11000 ft.
5. HAPE is the most common cause of death at altitude and usually occurs above 8000 ft.
6. Any respiratory distress at high altitude should be assumed as HAPE until proven otherwise.
7. Do not re-ascend until cleared by a medical officer.
8. Consider Acetazolamide (250mg PO BID or TID) prophylaxis beginning 24-48 hours out if mission planned at/above 10,000 feet or if drastic rapid ascent (air insertion) with medical officer approval.
9. Minimize the physical exertion of the casualty during descent using litters if possible.
10. Do not administer Diamox if suspected allergy to Sulfa products.

TACTICAL MEDICAL EMERGENCY PROTOCOLS

RANGER MEDIC Tactical Medical Emergency Protocols (TMEPs):

(Based on USSOCOM TMEPs dated 18 September 2006)

TMEP Properties: Relatively common, acute onset, life-threatening, adversely affects mission readiness, and/or rapid diagnosis and initial therapy can improve outcome.

TMEP Assumptions: Austere environment, absence of medical officer, patient is team member/coalition partner/detainee, evacuation is difficult, the problem may worsen if treatment is delayed, a medical officer will be contacted as soon as feasible, treatment is conducted IAW protocol, limited medications are available, and appropriate documentation will be conducted.

1. ACUTE (SURGICAL) ABDOMEN
2. ACUTE DENTAL PAIN
3. ACUTE MUSCULOSKELETAL BACK PAIN
4. ALLERGIC RHINITIS
5. ASTHMA (REACTIVE AIRWAY DISEASE)
6. BRONCHITIS
7. CELLULITIS
8. CHEST PAIN (CARDIAC ORIGIN SUSPECTED)
9. COMMON COLD
10. CONJUNCTIVITIS
11. CONSTIPATION
12. CONTACT DERMATITIS
13. CORNEAL ABRASION & CORNEAL ULCER
14. COUGH
15. CUTANEOUS ABSCESS
16. DEEP VENOUS THROMBOSIS (DVT)
17. DIARRHEA
18. EPIGLOTTITIS
19. EPISTAXIS
20. FUNGAL SKIN INFECTION
21. GASTROENTERITIS
22. GASTROESOPHAGEAL REFLUX DISEASE
23. HEADACHE
24. INGROWN TOENAIL
25. JOINT INFECTION
26. LACERATION
27. MALARIA
28. OTITIS EXTERNA
29. OTITIS MEDIA
30. PERITONSILLAR ABSCESS
31. PNEUMONIA
32. PULMONARY EMBOLISM
33. RENAL COLIC/KIDNEY STONES
34. SEPSIS/SEPTIC SHOCK
35. SMOKE INHALATION
36. SPRAINS & STRAINS
37. SUBUNGAL HEMATOMA
38. SYNCOPE
39. TESTICULAR PAIN
40. TONSILLOPHARYNGITIS
41. URINARY TRACT INFECTION (UTI)

1. ACUTE (SURGICAL) ABDOMEN

Definition: Common causes in young healthy adults include appendicitis, cholecystitis, pancreatitis, perforated ulcer, diverticulitis, or bowel obstruction

S/S: Severe, persistent or worsening abdominal pain; rigid abdomen, rebound tenderness, fever, anorexia, nausea/vomiting, absent bowel sounds, mild diarrhea if present

MGMT: 1. Keep patient NPO, except for water and meds, 2. NS IV at 150cc/hr, 3. Ertapenem (Invanz) or Ceftriaxone (Rocephin) 1gm IV/IM q24h, 4. Acetaminophen (Tylenol) 1000mg PO q6h prn pain, 5. Ondansetron (Zofran) 4mg IV over 2-5 minutes or IM bid or Phenergan (Promethazine) 12.5-25mg IV q4-6h for nausea/vomiting, 6. For severe pain, use Fentanyl Oral Lozenge (Actiq) 800mcg or Morphine Sulfate (MSO4) 5-10mg IV initially, then 5mg q30-60min prn pain, medicate to keep patient comfortable without loss of sensorium

Disposition: *Urgent* evacuation to facility with surgical capability

2. ACUTE DENTAL PAIN

Definition: Common causes are deep decay, fractures of tooth crown or root, or periapical abscess

S/S: Intermittent or continuous pain; heat or cold sensitivity; visibly broken tooth; severe pain on percussion; swelling or abscess

MGMT: 1. Acetaminophen (Tylenol) 1000mg PO q6h or Ibuprofen (Motrin) 800mg PO q8h prn pain, 2. If signs and symptoms of infection, Clindamycin (Cleocin) 300-450mg PO q6h or Amoxicillin/Clavulanic Acid (Augmentin) 500/125mg PO tid or 875/125mg PO bid or Ceftriaxone (Rocephin) 1gm IV/IM daily x 7d

Disposition: Evacuation usually not required; *Routine* evacuation if no response to therapy

3. ACUTE MUSCULOSKELETAL BACK PAIN

Definition: Back pain resulting from injury due to mechanical stress or functional demands

S/S: Acute or gradual onset of back pain that can be severe and debilitating; with or without radiation; aggravated by movement or certain positions, alleviated with rest; usually history of previous back pain

MGMT: 1. Acetaminophen (Tylenol) 500mg PO qid or Ibuprofen (Motrin) 800mg PO tid or Naproxen (Naprosyn) 500mg PO bid, 2. Cyclobenzaprine (Flexeril) 10mg PO tid or Methocarbamol (Robaxin) 1500mg PO qid, 3. Encourage fluid hydration, avoid bed rest, use ice pack if acute or heat pack if subacute, stretch as tolerated, 4. If acute and severe back pain and spasm, provide Ketorolac (Toradol) 15-30mg IV/IM and Diazepam (Valium) 5-10mg IV, and repeat once in 6-8h if needed, 5. Refer to *Spinal Trauma* protocol if abnormal neurological exam

Disposition: Evacuation usually not required; *Routine* evacuation if no response to therapy or acute lumbar disk disorder suspected; *Urgent* if neurological involvement (weakness, numbness, bowel or bladder dysfunction)

4. ALLERGIC RHINITIS

Definition: Inflammation of the nasal passages due to environmental allergy

S/S: Rhinorrhea with clear discharge, boggy or inflamed nasal mucosa, +/- nasal congestion, sneezing, nasal pruritis; +/- concurrent watery, pruritic, or red eyes; history of environmental allergy

MGMT: 1. Fluticasone (Flonase) 2 sprays in each nostril daily, 2. Antihistamines and decongestants prn, 3. Increase PO fluid intake

Disposition: Evacuation usually not required

5. ASTHMA (REACTIVE AIRWAY DISEASE)

Definition: Inflammatory disorder of the airway with bronchiolar hyper-responsiveness and narrowing of the distal airways; acute exacerbation seen with change in environment or level of allergen or irritant

S/S: Wheezing, dyspnea, chest tightness, decreased oxygen saturation, respiratory distress

MGMT: 1. Albuterol (Proventil) MDI 2-3 puffs q5min x 3 doses, 2. If no response, Epinephrine 0.5mg (0.5ml of 1:1000 solution) IM, repeat in 5-10 minutes if needed, 3. Saline lock, 4. Dexamethasone (Decadron) 10mg IV/IM, 5. Oxygen (if available), 6. Monitor with pulse ox, 7. If fever, chest pain, and cough, consider and treat as per *Pneumonia* protocol; if airway compromise refer to *Airway* protocol

Disposition: If adequate response, continue Albuterol q6h and Dexamethasone daily; if poor response, *Urgent* evacuation

6. BRONCHITIS

Definition: Inflammation of trachea, bronchi, and bronchioles resulting from upper respiratory tract infection (URI) or chemical irritant; viruses are the most common cause

S/S: Preceding URI symptoms, cough (initially unproductive, then productive), fatigue, +/- fever > 100.4, +/- dyspnea, injected pharynx

MGMT: 1. Hydrate, 2. Acetaminophen (Tylenol) 1000mg PO q6h prn fever, 3. Treat symptoms with antitussive, decongestants, expectorant, as needed, 3. Albuterol (Proventil) MDI 2 puffs q4-6hrs, 4. Smoking cessation, 5. If symptoms worsen or persist, consider and treat as per *Pneumonia* protocol

Disposition: Evacuation usually not required

7. CELLULITIS

Definition: Acute superficial spreading bacterial skin infection due to trauma or scratching of other lesions

S/S: Local warmth, pain, erythema, swelling with well-demarcated borders, +/- fever/chills, +/- lymphadenopathy; if rapidly spreading and very painful consider necrotizing fasciitis (life-threatening deep tissue infection) and treat per *Bacterial Sepsis* protocol

MGMT: 1. Acetaminophen (Tylenol) 1000mg PO q6h or Ibuprofen (Motrin) 800mg PO q8h prn pain, 2. Clindamycin (Cleocin) 300-450mg PO q6h or TMP-SMZ (Septra) DS PO bid or Moxifloxacin (Avelox) 400mg PO qd x 10 d, or Azithromycin (Zithromax) 250mg 2 tabs PO day 1 then 1 tab PO day 2-5, 3. Clean/dress wound, 4. Use marker to demarcate infection border, 5. Limit activity as feasible, 6. Reevaluate at least daily, 7. Identify and drain abscess if present, and 8. If severe or no response, use Ceftriaxone (Rocephin) or Ertapenem (Invanz) 1gm IV/IM qd and continue PO antibiotics

Disposition: *Priority* evacuation if infection fails to improve or worsens within 24-48hrs on antibiotics

8. CHEST PAIN (CARDIAC ORIGIN SUSPECTED)

Definition: Possible heart attack or myocardial infarction (MI)

S/S: Usually in patients over 40; history of hypertension, diabetes, smoking, elevated cholesterol, obesity; family history of MI at a young age; substernal pressure/squeezing chest pain +/- radiation to left arm or jaw, dyspnea, diaphoresis (sweating)

MGMT: 1. "MONA": Morphine Sulfate (MSO4) 4mg IV initially then 2mg IV q5-15min prn pain, Oxygen (if available), NTG (if available) 0.4mg SL initially, repeat q5min for total of 3 doses, Acetylsalicylic Acid (Aspirin) 325mg chew 2 tabs and swallow 2 tabs, 2. IV access, 3. Pulse oximetry and cardiac monitor (if available)

Disposition: *Urgent* evacuation on platform with ACLS personnel, medications, and equipment

9. COMMON COLD

Definition: Inflammation of nasal passages due to a respiratory virus

S/S: Nasal congestion, sneezing, sore throat, cough, hoarseness, malaise, headache, low-grade fever

MGMT: 1. Increase PO hydration, 2. Acetaminophen (Tylenol) 1000mg PO q6h, 3. Treat symptoms with decongestants, antihistamines, cough suppressants, and other symptomatic relief medications prn

Disposition: Evacuation usually not required

10. CONJUNCTIVITIS

Definition: Eye conjunctiva inflammation due to allergic, viral, or bacterial cause

S/S: All causes (burning, irritation, tearing); allergic (bilateral, serous or mucoid discharge, itching, redness); viral (unilateral, redness, watery discharge, conjunctival swelling, tender preauricular node, photophobia, foreign body sensation, associated URI); bacterial (unilateral, eye injection, mucopurulent or purulent discharge with morning crusting)

MGMT: 1. Discontinue contact lenses if applicable, 2. Cleanse with warm, wet wash cloth qid, 3. If allergy or viral, other than herpetic, artificial tears prn and Naphazolin/Pheniramine (Naphcon-A) 2 drops in affected eye qid, 4. If bacterial, Gatifloxacin (Zymar) 0.3% 1 drop in affected eye qid

Disposition: Evacuation usually not required

11. CONSTIPATION

Definition: Infrequent, hard, dry stools

S/S: Infrequent, hard, dry stools with possible pain/straining with defecation, abdominal fullness, and poorly localized cramping abdominal pain; if pain becomes severe with N/V and lack of flatus or stools consider bowel obstruction; if acute onset, severe pain, rigid board-like abdomen, rebound or point tenderness, and/or fever, consider other disorders (appendicitis, bowel obstruction, cholecystitis, diverticulitis, pancreatitis, and ulcer) and treat as per *Acute (Surgical) Abdomen* protocol

MGMT: 1. Increase PO fluids and fiber – fruits, bran, vegetables, 2. Docusate (Colace) 100mg PO bid, 3. Acetaminophen (Tylenol) 1000mg PO q6h prn pain (*no narcotics – they cause constipation!*), 4. If impacted or no response give 500cc NS enema per rectum (lubricate IV tubing), 5. If continued no response, perform digital rectal exam (DRE) and digital disimpaction, 6. Consider parasitic infection

Disposition: *Routine* evacuation if no response to treatment; *Urgent* evacuation if acute abdomen

12. CONTACT DERMATITIS

Definition: Skin reaction to external substance (plants, metals, chemicals, topical medications)

S/S: Acute onset of skin erythema and pruritis; may see edema, papules, vesicles, bullae, and possible discharge and crusting; evaluate and monitor for secondary bacterial infection and treat per *Cellulitis* protocol if suspected; consider insect bite and fungal infection in differential diagnosis

MGMT: 1. Remove offending agent and evaluate pattern, 2. Wash area with soap and water, 3. Change and/or wash clothes, 4. Topical cold wet compress AAA, 5. Topical calamine lotion AAA, 6. Topical high-potency steroid cream AAA qid (low-potency on face), 7. Diphenhydramine (Benadryl) 25-50mg PO qid prn pruritis, 8. If severe, Solu-Medrol 125 mg IM x 1; or Dexamethasone (Decadron) 10mg IM daily x 5 d; or Prednisone 60mg PO daily x 5 d burst or taper dose down every 3 days for a 14-21 day course

Disposition: *Priority* evacuation if severe, eye or mouth involved, or > 50% BSA involved

13. CORNEAL ABRASION & CORNEAL ULCER

Definition: A traumatic disruption of the epithelial covering of the cornea; three major concerns: intense eye pain, corneal ulcer (vision-threatening infection), and potential for ruptured globe

S/S: History of eye trauma or contact lens wear with eye pain; redness, tearing, blurred vision, light sensitivity, positive fluorescein stain/cobalt blue light (bright yellow area on cornea); increasing pain and white or gray spot on cornea with tangential penlight indicative of corneal ulcer; blood in anterior chamber, bulging subconjunctival hemorrhage (chemosis), and peaked pupil indicative of ruptured globe; if history of LASIK, consider flap dislocation

MGMT: 1. Examine eye, to include eyelid eversion, and remove any foreign body, 2. Gatifloxacin (Zymar) 0.3% 1 drop in affected eye qid until after 24h fluorescein negative (q2h if corneal ulcer), 3. If available, Tetracaine 0.5% 2 drops in affected eye for pain (do not give bottle to patient), 4. Acetaminophen (Tylenol) 1000mg PO q6h prn pain, 5. No patching, 6. Reduce light exposure/stay indoors/wear sunglasses as feasible, 7. Monitor daily with fluorescein

Disposition: *Routine* evacuation if not improving; *Priority* evacuation if corneal ulcer; *Urgent* evacuation and eye shield if ruptured globe suspected; *Urgent* evacuation if LASIK flap dislocation

14. COUGH

Definition: Usually viral etiology, but may occur with HAPE, pneumonia, GERD, and smoking history

S/S: Cough with or without scant sputum production, often accompanied by other URI S/S (sore throat, rhinorrhea, post-nasal drip)

MGMT: 1. Treat symptomatically if history and physical exam do not suggest pneumonia, 2. Increase PO hydration, 3. Avoid respiratory irritants (smoke, aerosols, etc), 4. Benzonatate (Tessalon perles) 100mg PO tid or Dextromethorphan (Robitussin DM) 30mg PO bid prn cough, 5. Albuterol (Proventil) MDI 3-4 puffs q4h can help if cough continues; Treat per *Pneumonia* protocol if fever, chest pain, dyspnea, colored sputum (green, dark yellow, red-tinged)

Disposition: Evacuation usually not required

15. CUTANEOUS ABSCESS

Definition: Cutaneous abscess

S/S: Focal pain, erythema, warmth, tenderness, swelling, and fluctuance

MGMT: 1. Clindamycin (Cleocin) 300-450mg PO q6h or TMP-SMZ (Septra) DS PO bid or Moxifloxacin (Avelox) 400mg PO qd x 10 d, or Azithromycin (Zithromax) 250mg PO 2 tabs PO day 1 then 1 tab PO day 2-5, 2. I&D if not on eyelid, face, or neck (sterilize site with betadine, anesthetize with 1% Lidocaine, incise parallel to skin tension lines with scalpel and make opening large enough to allow purulence to drain, pack with iodoform gauze or nu-gauze, cover with loose bandage; check, redress, and wick q12-24hrs); Do not suture, drainage is the key to treatment!

Disposition: Evacuation usually not required; If condition worsens treat per *Cellulitis* protocol and evacuate as *Priority*

16. DEEP VENOUS THROMBOSIS (DVT)

Definition: Potentially life-threatening condition in which a clot is present in the large veins of a leg and may dislodge and localize in the pulmonary system, a pulmonary embolism (PE)

S/S: History of recent trauma, air travel, altitude exposure, birth control pills, or family history of DVT; pain, swelling, and warmth seen in legs (usually calf), but may occur in any deep vein; palpable venous "cord"; pain with passive stretching or dorsiflexion of the foot

MGMT: 1. Acetylsalicylic acid (Aspirin) 325mg PO q4-6h, 2. Immobilize and do not allow to walk on affected extremity, 3. Monitor with pulse oximetry (sudden decrease suggests PE), if tachypnea, tachycardia, respiratory distress, and chest pain develop, treat per *Pulmonary Embolism* protocol

Disposition: *Priority* evacuation; *Urgent* if PE suspected

17. DIARRHEA

Definition: Loose bowel movements (BM); abrupt onset in healthy individuals usually related to infectious cause (viral, bacterial, parasitic)

S/S: Loose or watery BMs, +/- blood or mucous, +/- fever, abdominal cramping, discomfort, and/or distension; possible S/S of dehydration (decreased and/or dark urine output, lightheadedness, headache, dry mucosa, poor skin turgor, degradation in performance)

MGMT: 1. Replace lost fluids and electrolytes, PO if tolerated, if not then IV LR or NS, 2. Loperamide (Imodium) 4mg PO initially, then 2mg after every loose BM, max of 16mg/day, 3. If diarrhea persists > 24 hrs, give Azithromycin (Zithromax) 500mg or Moxifloxacin (Avelox) 400mg PO qd or Ciprofloxacin (Cipro) 500mg PO bid x 3d, 4. If diarrhea > 3 days, treat as Giardia or Amebiasis with Tinidazole (Tindamax) 2gm PO qd or Metronidazole (Flagyl) 500mg PO tid x 3d

Disposition: Evacuation usually not required, if dehydration despite therapy or antibiotic-related diarrhea, evacuate as *Priority*. Grossly bloody stools or circulatory compromise require *Urgent* evacuation

18. EPIGLOTTITIS

Definition: Inflammation of the epiglottis

S/S: Sore throat, difficulty speaking and swallowing, drooling, respiratory distress, erythematous pharynx; first symptom of severe sore throat progresses to epiglottal swelling and potential for airway obstruction

MGMT: 1. Place patient in sitting or comfortable position, 2. IV access, 3. Ceftriaxone (Rocephin) 2gm IV/IM q12h, 4. Dexamethasone (Decadron) 8mg IV/IM x 1, 5. Pulse oximetry, 6. Oxygen if available, 7. Do not manipulate airway unless required, let the patient protect his own airway, 8. If definitive airway is needed, make one attempt at intubation, and if failed, perform a cricothyroidotomy

Disposition: *Urgent* evacuation

19. EPISTAXIS

Definition: Nosebleed

S/S: Nosebleed, often with previous history of nosebleeds; common at altitude and in desert environments due to mucosal drying; may be anterior or posterior; posterior epistaxis may be difficult to stop and may cause respiratory distress due to blood flowing into airway; posterior epistaxis is more commonly seen in older hypertensive patients

MGMT: 1. Clear airway by having patient sit up and lean forward, 2. Oxymetazoline (Afrin) 2-3 sprays intranasally and pinch anterior area of nose firmly for full 10 minutes without releasing pressure, 3. If bleeding continues, insert Afrin-soaked nasal sponge along floor of nasal cavity, remove 30 minutes after bleeding is controlled, and apply Mupirocin (Bactroban) bid-tid, 5. If severe nosebleed and bleeding continues, initiate saline lock or NS TKO and consider inserting 14 French Foley catheter intranasally for 72h, 6. If packing and/or catheter required for > 12h, treat with Moxifloxacin (Avelox) 400mg PO qd

Disposition: Evacuation not required for mild, anterior, and resolving epistaxis; *Priority* evacuation for severe epistaxis not responding to therapy or if Foley used

20. FUNGAL SKIN INFECTION

Definition: Fungal skin infection

S/S: Scaling plaques, erythema, pruritic, slow spreading, irregular or circumferential borders; often initially diagnosed as contact dermatitis but gets worse with steroid cream; most common sites of infection are feet ("athlete's foot" or tinea pedis), groin ("jock itch" or tinea cruris), scalp (tinea capitus), and torso or extremities ("ring worm" or tinea corporis); differential diagnosis includes eczema, insect bites, cellulitis, and contact dermatitis

MGMT: 1. Antifungal cream AAA tid until one week after lesion resolves, 2. In moderate to severe cases, use Fluconazole (Diflucan) 150 mg PO qwk x 2 wks or Ketoconazole (Nizoral) 200-400 mg PO qd or Terbinafine (Lamisil) 250 mg PO qd

Disposition: Evacuation not required

21. GASTROENTERITIS

Definition: Usually due to an acute viral infection of the GI tract, but bacteria or parasite infections are common in deployed environments

S/S: Sudden onset of N/V/D, abdominal cramping, +/- fever

MGMT: 1. Loperamide (Imodium) 4mg PO initially, then 2mg after every loose BM, max of 16mg/day (do not use if bloody stools or fevers), 2. If nausea/vomiting, Promethazine (Phenergan) 12.5-25mg PO/IM/IV or Ondansetron (Zofran) 4mg IV over 2-5 minutes or IM bid, 3. If diarrhea persists > 24 hrs, give Azithromycin (Zithromax) 500mg PO daily or Moxifloxacin (Avelox) 400mg PO daily or Ciprofloxacin (Cipro) 500mg PO bid; Azithromycin new primary agent due to emerging quinolone resistance among enteropathogenic E. coli, 4. PO hydrate with ORS, Cyralyte, Gatorade, Powerade, and water, 5. 1-2 liters NS or LR IV if PO not tolerated and titrate fluid intake to regain normal urine frequency and color, good skin turgor, and moist mucous membranes, 6. If diarrhea > 3 days treat as Giardia or Amebiasis treat with Tinidazole (Tindamax) 2gm PO qd or Metronidazole (Flagyl) 500mg PO tid x 3d

Disposition: Evacuation usually not required; *Priority* evacuation if dehydration despite therapy or antibiotic-related diarrhea; *Urgent* evacuation if grossly bloody stools or circulatory compromise

22. GASTROESOPHAGEAL REFLUX DISEASE (GERD)

Definition: Reflux of gastroduodenal contents into esophagus due to improper lower esophageal sphincter relaxation

S/S: Heartburn, regurgitation, dysphagia

MGMT: 1. Avoid high-fat food, onion, tomato chocolate, peppermint, citrus, tobacco, coffee, alcohol, 2. Elevate head on bed when sleeping and do not eat just before bedtime, 3. Ranitidine (Zantac) 150mg or Cimetidine (Tagamet) 400mg PO bid, or Rabeprazole (Aciphex) or Omeprazole (Prilosec) 20mg PO qd or bid, 4. If on Doxycycline for malaria chemoprophylaxis, take the doxy early in the day with a meal

Disposition: Evacuation usually not required

23. HEADACHE

Definition: Headache

S/S: Episodic or chronic, secondary to stressor; unilateral or bilateral, localized or general, dull or band-like, with or without nausea/vomiting; sometimes associated with caffeine withdrawal, neck muscle tightness, teeth grinding; if atypical, check for elevated blood pressure, fever, neck rigidity, visual symptoms, photophobia, mental status changes, neurological weakness, rash, and hydration and treat per appropriate protocol

MGMT: 1. If caffeine withdrawal, consider caffeine 100-200mg (1-2 cups coffee), 2. Acetaminophen (Tylenol) 1000mg PO q6hrs or Ibuprofen (Motrin) 800mg PO tid or Naproxen (Naprosyn) 500mg PO bid, 3. If nausea/vomiting, Promethazine (Phenergan) 12.5-25mg PO/IM/IV or Ondansetron (Zofran) 4mg IV over 2-5 minutes or IM bid, 4. If dehydration suspected, PO or IV hydration, 5. If new-onset migraine suspected, refer to a medical officer; usually benign, but consider AMS, intracranial bleed, or meningitis

Disposition: Evacuation usually not required; *Urgent* evacuation if acute headache with fever, severe nausea/vomiting, mental status changes, focal neuro signs, or preceding seizures, LOC, or history of "it's the worst headache of my life"

24. INGROWN TOENAIL

Definition: Usually big toe; due to trimming nails in curved fashion, nail deformity, tight fitting shoes, and rotational toe deformity

S/S: Pain, edema, erythema, hyperkeratosis at lateral nail fold; pressure on nail margin increases pain

MGMT: 1. Partial toenail removal: clean site with soap, water, and betadine; local anesthesia through digital block using 1% lidocaine without epinephrine; apply tourniquet at base; remove lateral ¼ of nail toward cuticle, using sharp scissors; separate nail from the underlying matrix and remove; curette posterior and lateral nail grooves to remove debris; rub matrix with silver nitrate stick; apply Mupirocin (Bactroban) and cover with nonadherent and dry sterile dressings; wash, clean, recheck wound and change dressing daily, 2. Acetaminophen (Tylenol) 1000mg PO q6h prn pain, 3. Systemic antibiotics usually not needed, however use Moxifloxacin (Avelox) 400mg PO qd x 10d or Azithromycin (Zithromax) 250mg 2 tabs PO day 1 then 1 tab PO day 2-5 if in tactical setting or infection (increasing pain, redness, and swelling)

Disposition: Evacuation usually not required

25. JOINT INFECTION

Definition: Bacterial joint infection, septic arthritis, septic joint; may result from penetrating trauma

S/S: Fever and red swollen painful joint; pain with axial load; inability to straighten joint; history of animal or human bite, needle aspiration of joint effusion, gonorrhea

MGMT: 1. Immobilize joint, 2. Ertapenem (Invanz) 1gm IV/IM daily or Ceftriaxone (Rocephin) 2gm IV/IM bid, 3. Acetaminophen (Tylenol) 1000mg PO q6h or Ibuprofen (Motrin) 800mg PO tid prn pain

Disposition: *Priority* evacuation

26. LACERATION

Definition: Skin laceration

S/S: Simple uncomplicated laceration of skin without involvement of deeper structures

MGMT: 1: Irrigate and clean wound thoroughly, 2. Prepare area in sterile fashion, 3. Provide local anesthesia with 1% Lidocaine, 4. Close with absorbable suture, non-absorbable suture, dermabond, or steri-strips as dependent on depth of wound, 5. If dirty wound or environment, Clindamycin (Cleocin) 300-450mg PO q6h or TMP-SMZ (Septra) DS PO bid or Moxifloxacin (Avelox) 400mg PO qd x 10 d, 6. Check tetanus status and treat as needed; do not suture if wound is > 12 h old (> 24 h on face), or if puncture/bite wound

Disposition: Evacuation usually not required

27. MALARIA

Definition: Protozoan infection transmitted by Anopheles mosquito; prevention through personal protective measures is the key (anti-malarial meds, DEET, permethrin, minimize exposed skin)

S/S: History of travel to malaria-endemic area, non-compliance with anti-malarial meds and/or personal protective measures; malaise, fatigue, and myalgia followed by recurrent episodes of fevers, chills, rigors, profuse sweats, headache, backache, nausea, vomiting, diarrhea; tachycardia, orthostatic hypotension, tender hepatomegaly, moderate splenomegaly, and delirium

MGMT: 1. If available, attempt to diagnosis with lab (serial blood smears and rapid test); if unavailable and malaria suspected, empirically treat with Mefloquine (Larium) 750mg PO initially followed by 500mg PO 12h later or Malarone 4 tabs PO daily with food x 3 days or Chloroquine 10mg/kg base PO x 2 days then 5mg/kg PO x 1 day (concomitant Primaquine may also be required) 2. Acetaminophen (Tylenol) 1000mg PO q6h prn fever

Disposition: *Routine* evacuation for uncomplicated cases; *Urgent* evacuation if cerebral, pulmonary, or vital sign instability

28. OTITIS EXTERNA

Definition: Bacterial or fungal infection of external ear canal, "swimmer's ear"

S/S: Ear pain and pain with passive ear movement; swelling, erythema, pruritis in area; possible exudate and erythema in ear canal, decreased auditory acuity, sensation of fullness and moisture in ear

MGMT: 1. Gatifloxacin (Zymar) 0.3% 4 drops in affected ear q2h while awake and laying on side for at least 5 minutes; ophthalmic used to minimize meds carried, but if available, Cortisporin otic 5 drops tid-qid until 48h after symptoms resolve, 2. Sterile dry dressing wick into ear canal, 3. (Acetaminophen) Tylenol 1000mg PO q6h prn pain, 4. If no response or worsens, use Moxifloxacin (Avelox) 400mg PO daily x 10d or Azithromycin (Zithromax) 250mg 2 tabs PO day 1 then 1 tab PO day 2-5 , 5. No internal hearing protection until resolution

Disposition: Evacuation usually not required; *Priority* evacuation if "malignant" otitis externa (Severe headache, otorrhea (purulent ear drainage), cranial nerve palsy)

29. OTITIS MEDIA

Definition: Eustachian tube dysfunction, viral infection, or bacterial infection of middle ear

S/S: Ear pain, +/- fever, decreased hearing, sensation of ear fullness; erythema and bulging of TM are hallmark signs, increased pressure may cause TM rupture and discharge; often noted with accompanying URI symptoms, recent air travel, or recent ascent to altitude

MGMT: 1. Acetaminophen (Tylenol) 1000mg PO q6h or Ibuprofen (Motrin) 800mg PO tid prn pain, 2. Oxymetazoline (Afrin) nasal spray 2 squirts per nostril bid (max 3 days), 3. If grossly apparent, or no resolution in 1-2 d, add antibiotics: Moxifloxacin (Avelox) 400mg PO daily or TMP-SMZ (Septra) DS PO bid x 10d or Azithromycin (Zithromax) 250mg 2 tabs PO day 1 then 1 tab PO day 2-5

Disposition: Evacuation usually not required; *Routine* evacuation for TM rupture or complicated cases not responding to therapy

30. PERITONSILLAR ABSCESS

Definition: Infection with abscess formation and pus collection between anterior and posterior tonsillar pillars, usually following acute episode of tonsillopharyngitis

S/S: Extreme sore throat or neck pain, dysphagia, dysphonia, fever, erythema, edema, asymmetry of oropharynx with deviation of uvula

MGMT: 1. Clindamycin (Cleocin) 300-450mg PO q6h or Amoxicillin/Clavulanic Acid (Augmentin) 500/125mg PO tid or 875/125mg PO bid or Ceftriaxone (Rocephin) 1gm IV/IM daily x 7d, 2. Acetaminophen (Tylenol) 1000mg PO q6h or Ibuprofen (Motrin) 800mg PO tid prn pain/fever, 3. If unresolving or worsening symptoms to include airway obstruction, the patient must be evacuated for needle aspiration or I&D (caution must be used to avoid carotid artery perforation)

Disposition: *Routine* evacuation; *Priority* evacuation if airway obstruction

31. PNEUMONIA

Definition: Acute lung infection due to virus, mycoplasma, or other bacteria

S/S: Fever, chills, productive cough (dark yellow, green, red tinged), chest pain, malaise, wheezes, rhonchi and/or rales, decreased breath sounds, dyspnea, tachypnea, SOB

MGMT: 1. If mild to moderate, Azithromycin (Zithromax) 250mg 2 tabs PO day 1 then 1 tab PO day 2-5 or Moxifloxacin (Avelox) 400mg PO daily x 5d or Doxycycline 100mg PO bid x 10 d; If severe, start with Ceftriaxone (Rocephin) 2gm q12h or Ertapenem (Invanz) daily IM/IV, then oral antibiotic regimen, 2. Acetaminophen (Tylenol) 1000mg PO q6h prn pain/fever, 3. Albuterol (Proventil) MDI 2 puffs qid prn wheezing, 4. PO hydration, 5. Pulse oximetry, 6. Oxygen if hypoxic, 7. If at altitude > 8000 ft, descend 1,500 – 3,000 feet; differential diagnosis should include HAPE, PE, and pneumothorax

Disposition: *Priority* evacuation; *Urgent* evacuation for severe dyspnea

32. PULMONARY EMBOLUS (PE)

Definition: Usually occurs when leg DVT dislodges and enters pulmonary arterial circulation

S/S: Acute onset of dyspnea, tachypnea, tachycardia, localized chest pain, anxiety, diaphoresis (sweating), decreased oxygen saturation, full breath sounds with no wheezing, no prominent cough, and low-grade fever; usually proceeded by DVT with lower extremity pain, swelling, and tenderness with history of trauma, air travel, or long periods in sitting positions

MGMT: 1. Monitor with pulse oximetry and provide oxygen (if available), 2. Acetylsalicylic Acid (Aspirin) 325mg chew 2 tabs, 3. Morphine Sulfate (MSO4) 4mg IV initially then 2mg IV q5-15min prn pain, 4. Consider Myocardial Infarction and treat as per *Chest Pain* protocol, 5. If at altitude > 8,000ft, descend 1500–3000 ft as per *HAPE* protocol

Disposition: *Urgent* evacuation

33. RENAL COLIC / KIDNEY STONES

Definition: Spasmodic kidney pain typically caused by kidney stone; may be associated with preceding lower urinary tract infection (UTI) or obstruction

S/S: Back pain, flank pain, nausea/vomiting, CVAT, fever, chills, frequency, urgency, dysuria

MGMT: 1. Moxifloxacin (Avelox) 400mg PO daily x 7d or Azithromycin (Zithromax) 250mg 2 tabs PO day 1 then 1 tab PO day 2-5 ; If PO not tolerated, Ceftriaxone (Rocephin) 2gm q12h or Ertapenem (Invanz) daily IM/IV, 2. Acetaminophen (Tylenol) 1000mg PO q6h or Ibuprofen (Motrin) 800mg PO tid prn pain, 3. Promethazine (Phenergan) 12.5-25mg IV or Ondansetron (Zofran) 4mg IV over 2 to 5 minutes or IM bid prn nausea/vomiting, 5. PO hydration, NS or LR IV at 250cc/hr if unable to tolerate PO, 6. monitor urine output

Disposition: *Priority* evacuation; may progress to life-threatening systemic infection and septic shock

34. SEPSIS/SEPTIC SHOCK

Definition: Severe life-threatening bacterial blood infection, rapid onset, death may occur within 4-6 hrs without antibiotic therapy

S/S: Hypotension, fever, chills, tachycardia, altered mental status, dyspnea, possible purpuric skin rash

MGMT: 1. IV or IO access, 2. Ertapenem (Invanz) 1gm IV/IM daily or Ceftriaxone (Rocephin) 2gm IV/IM daily, q12hrs if considering meningitis, 3. If hypotensive, give 2L NS or LR bolus (if unavailable, give 1L Hextend), 4. If hypotension continues, give Epinephrine (1:1000) 0.5mg IM, repeat 2L NS bolus, and titrate fluids to maintain SBP > 90 mmHg (NOTE: May require 10L crystalloid fluids within first 24 hrs), 5. Monitor urine output with goal of 30cc/hr (insert foley catheter if available), 6. Monitor mental status and be prepared to manage airway

Disposition: *Urgent* evacuation

35. SMOKE INHALATION

Definition: Common after closed space exposure to fire; consider airway burns, carbon monoxide poisoning, other toxin inhalation, and need for hyperbaric oxygen

S/S: History of smoke exposure, burns, singed nares, facial burns, coughing, respiratory distress

MGMT: 1. Refer to *Airway Management* protocol and consider early cricothyroidotomy or intubation, 2. Albuterol (Proventil) MDI 2-4 puffs q4-6h, 3. Dexamethasone (Decadron) 10mg IV/IM daily x 2 days, 4. Oxygen if available, 5. Limit exertion and activity

Disposition: *Priority* evacuation if significant inhalation; *Urgent* evacuation if respiratory distress

36. SPRAINS & STRAINS

Definition: Sprain or strain of musculoskeletal structures

S/S: Swelling, pain, erythema, ecchymosis, tenderness, decreased range of motion

MGMT: 1. "RICE" (Rest, Ice, Compression, Elevation), 2. Orthosis/splint/crutches for pain relief and stability, 3. Ibuprofen (Motrin) 800mg PO tid or Naproxen (Naprosyn) 500mg PO bid prn pain, 4. If no fracture, initiate rehab immediately; active range of motion exercises as tolerated; encourage weight bearing as tolerated; suspect occult fracture if no improvement within one week

Disposition: Evacuation usually not required

37. SUBUNGAL HEMATOMA

Definition: Collection of blood under the nail; typically occurs after trauma to fingernail or toenail

S/S: Pain and purplish-black discoloration under nail

MGMT: 1. Decompress nail with large gauge needle introduced through nail over discolored area with a gentle but sustained rotating motion until underlying blood and pressure is relieved; gentle pressure to the nail immediately after the procedure may evacuate additional blood, 2. Acetaminophen (Tylenol) 1000mg PO q6h prn pain, 3. Tape/splint if fracture suspected

Disposition: Evacuation usually not required

38. SYNCOPE

Definition: Orthostatic hypotension; fainting as a result of vasovagal response

S/S: Sudden and brief loss of consciousness, without seizures, and with return to normal mentation

MGMT: 1. Supportive care; place in supine position and ensure airway is open, should regain consciousness within a few seconds, if not: 2. Check blood glucose, and use oral glucose gel or sugar sublingually, 3. If no response, consider heat injury, anaphylaxis, cardiac, and pulmonary etiologies and treat as per protocol, 4. Check vitals and pulse oximetry, 5. Oxygen if available, 6. Cardiac monitoring

Disposition: Evacuation usually not required; unless other diagnosis or symptoms continue/recur

39. TESTICULAR PAIN

Definition: Testicular pain due to torsion, epididymitis, orchitis, STDs, hernias, masses, and trauma

S/S: Torsion: sudden onset of pain, pain-induced nausea/vomiting, swelling, abnormal lie of testicle, symptoms increase with elevation, associated with activity; Epididymitis: gradual onset of worsening pain, +/- fever, +/- dysuria, +/- trauma

MGMT: 1. If torsion suspected, manually detorse by rotating outward "open the book", if pain increases attempt once to rotate in opposite direction, 2. If other cause suspected, consider and treat as per *Urinary Tract Infection* protocol and treat pain as per *Pain Management* protocol

Disposition: *Urgent* evacuation for unrelieved torsion; *Priority* evacuation for relieved torsion; for other causes consider evacuation as symptoms warrant or treatment fails

40. TONSILLOPHARYNGITIS

Definition: Acute bacterial or viral infection/inflammation of the pharynx, ¼ caused by Group A Beta Hemolytic Streptococcus (GABHS)

S/S: Sore throat, enlarged and edematous tonsils, erythema and exudates, palatal petechiae, anterior cervical lymphadenopathy; fever > 102.5 suggestive of bacterial cause; throat culture is most accurate test for GABHS

MGMT: 1. Salt water gargles, 2. Acetaminophen (Tylenol) 1000mg PO q6h, 3. If bacterial suspected, Azithromycin (Zithromax) 500mg PO daily x 3 days, 4) Observe and treat as per *Peritonsillar Abscess* protocol as required, 5) Consider concurrent infection with Ebstein-Barr virus (Infectious Mononucleosis)

Disposition: Evacuation usually not required

41. URINARY TRACT INFECTION (UTI)

Definition: Infection of urinary tract; more common in females, tactical setting, dehydration, kidney stones

S/S: Frequency, urgency, dysuria; no CVAT/back/flank pain, no fever; possible cloudy malodorous or dark urine, suprapubic discomfort

MGMT: 1. Moxifloxacin (Avelox) 400mg PO daily x 3d **_and_** Azithromycin (Zithromax) 1000mg x 1 dose (to treat for STDs), 2. Acetaminophen (Tylenol) 1000mg q6h prn pain, 3. PO hydration, 4. If fever, CVAT, back pain, or flank pain, suspect and treat per *Renal Colic* protocol

Disposition: Evacuation usually not required; *Routine* evacuation if symptoms worsen or no resolution

SECTION THREE

RMED PHARMACOLOGY
SECTION I

"PROFICIENT AND ALWAYS CARRIED"

PHARMACOLOGY SECTION I: "PROFICIENT AND ALWAYS CARRIED"

1.	ACETAMINOPHEN (TYLENOL)	325-650 mg PO q4-6h prn (max: 4 g/d)
2.	DEXAMETHASONE	0.25–4 mg PO bid-qid; 8–16 mg IM/IV q1–3wks
3.	DIAZEPAM (VALIUM)	2-10 mg PO tid-qid; 5-10 mg slow IV push
4.	DIPHENHYDRAMINE (BENADRYL)	25-50 mg IV/IM/PO q4-6h
5.	EPINEPHRINE	0.1–0.5 mL SC/IM q10–15min (1:1000 soln = 1mg/1ml)
6.	ERTAPENEM (INVANZ)	1g IV/IM q24h
7.	FENTANYL ORAL LOZENGES (ACTIQ)	400-800 mcg (max: 1600 mcg/d)
8.	GATIFLOXACIN (TEQUIN)	400 mg IV/PO daily
9.	HETASTARCH (HEXTEND)	500–1000 mL IV
10.	IBUPROFEN (MOTRIN, ADVIL)	400–800 mg PO tid-qid (max: 3200 mg/d)
11.	KETOROLAC (TORADOL)	15-30 mg IV/IM q6h
12.	LIDOCAINE (XYLOCAINE)	Infiltration 0.5%–2% injection
13.	MELOXICAM (MOBIC)	7.5–15 mg PO daily
14.	MORPHINE SULFATE (MSO4)	5–15mg slow IV push, titrate to pain
15.	MOXIFLOXACIN (AVELOX)	400 mg PO/IV daily
16.	NALOXONE (NARCAN)	0.4–2.0 mg IV, repeat q2–3min up to 10 mg prn
17.	PROMETHAZINE (PHENERGAN)	12.5-25 mg PO/IM/IV q4-6h prn
18.	SODIUM CHLORIDE, 0.9% (NS)	500–1000 mL IV; 5-50 mL IV for med dilution or flush

1. ACETAMINOPHEN (TYLENOL)

Class: CNS agent – non-narcotic, analgesic, antipyretic

Action: Analgesia action possibly through peripheral nervous system; fever reduction through direct action on hypothalamus heat-regulating center resulting in peripheral vasodilation, sweating, and dissipation of heat; has minimal effect on platelet aggregation, bleeding time, and gastric bleeding

Dose: 325–650 mg PO q4–6h (max: 4 g/d)

Indications: For mild to moderate pain management, headache, fever reduction

Contraindications: Acetaminophen hypersensitivity; use with alcohol; pregnancy category B

Adverse Effects: Negligible with recommended dose; rash; acute poisoning: anorexia, nausea, vomiting, dizziness, lethargy, diaphoresis, chills, epigastric or abdominal pain, diarrhea; hepatotoxicity: elevation of liver function tests; hypoglycemia, hepatic coma, acute renal failure; chronic ingestion: neutropenia, pancytopenia, leukopenia, thrombocytopenic purpura, renal damage

Interactions: Cholestyramine may decrease absorption; barbiturates, carbamazepine, phenytoin, rifampin, and excessive alcohol use may increase potential for hepatotoxicity

2. DEXAMETHASONE

Class: Hormones and synthetic substitutes – steroid; adrenocorticoid; glucocorticoid

Action: Long-acting synthetic adrenocorticoid with intense glucocorticoid activity and minimal mineralocorticoid activity; Antiinflammatory and immunosuppression properties; prevents accumulation of inflammatory cells at sites of infection; inhibits phagocytosis, lysosomal enzyme release, and synthesis of selected chemical mediators of inflammation; reduces capillary dilation and permeability

Dose: 0.25–4 mg PO bid-qid; 8–16 mg IM/IV q1–3wks

Indications: For inflammatory conditions, allergic states, and cerebral edema

Contraindications: Systemic fungal infection, acute infections, tuberculosis, vaccinia, varicella, live virus vaccines (to patient, family members), amebiasis; pregnancy category C

Adverse Effects: Euphoria, insomnia, convulsions, increased ICP, vertigo, headache, psychic disturbances; CHF, hypertension, edema; hyperglycemia; cushingoid state; hirsutism; cataracts, increased IOP, glaucoma, exophthalmos; peptic ulcer or perforation, abdominal distension, nausea, increased appetite, heartburn, dyspepsia, pancreatitis, bowel perforation, oral candidiasis; muscle weakness, loss of muscle mass, vertebral compression fracture, pathologic fracture of long bones, tendon rupture; acne, impaired wound healing, petechiae, ecchymoses, diaphoresis, dermatitis, hypo- or hyperpigmentation, skin atrophy

Interactions: May inhibit antibody response to vaccines and toxoids

3. DIAZEPAM (VALIUM) - CONTROLLED SUBSTANCE: SCHEDULE IV

Class: CNS agent – benzodiazepine; anticonvulsant; anxiolytic

Action: Anticonvulsant and antianxiety psychotherapeutic drug with action at both limbic and subcortical levels of CNS; increases total sleep time, but shortens REM and stage 4 sleep

Dose: 2-10 mg po tid-qid; 5-10 mg slow IV push, repeat in 3-4h

Indications: For anxiety, seizures, skeletal muscle spasm relief; also used as an amnesic, for treatment of restless leg syndrome, acute alcohol withdrawal, and is the drug of choice for status epilepticus

Contraindications: Shock, coma, alcohol intoxication, depressed vital signs; acute narrow-angle glaucoma, untreated open-angle glaucoma; MAOIs; pregnancy category D

Adverse Effects: Throat and chest pain; drowsiness, fatigue, ataxia, confusion, paradoxic rage, dizziness, vertigo, amnesia, vivid dreams, headache, slurred speech, tremor; EEG changes, tardive dyskinesia; hypotension, tachycardia, edema, cardiovascular collapse; blurred vision, diplopia, nystagmus; xerostomia, nausea, constipation, hepatic dysfunction; incontinence, urinary retention, gynecomastia (prolonged use); hiccups, coughing, laryngospasm; venous thrombosis, phlebitis

Interactions: Alcohol, CNS depressants, anticonvulsants, and herbals (kava kava, valerian) potentiate CNS depression; cimetidine increases levels and toxicity; may decrease effects of levodopa; may increase phenytoin levels; smoking decreases sedative and antianxiety effects

4. DIPHENHYDRAMINE (BENADRYL)

Class: ENT agent – H_1-blocker; antihistamine

Action: H_1-receptor antagonist and antihistamine as it competes for H_1-receptor sites on effector cells; significant central anticholinergic activity as it prolongs action of dopamine by inhibiting its reuptake and storage, thus decreasing parkinsonism and drug-induced extrapyramidal symptoms

Dose: 25-50 mg IV/IM/PO q4-6h

Indications: For allergic conditions, treatment or prevention of motion sickness, vertigo, blood or plasma reactions, treatment of Parkinsonism and drug-induced extrapyramidal reactions; also used with epinephrine for anaphylaxis, as a cough suppressant, a sedative-hypnotic, and for intractable insomnia

Contraindications: Antihistamine hypersensitivity; lower respiratory tract symptoms, asthma; narrow-angle glaucoma; prostatic hypertrophy, bladder neck obstruction; GI obstruction; pregnancy category C

Adverse Effects: Drowsiness, dizziness, headache, fatigue, disturbed coordination, tingling, heaviness and weakness of hands, tremors, euphoria, nervousness, restlessness, insomnia; confusion; excitement, fever, palpitation, tachycardia, hypo- or hypertension, cardiovascular collapse, tinnitus, vertigo, dry nose, throat, nasal stuffiness; blurred vision, diplopia, photosensitivity, dry eyes, dry mouth, nausea, epigastric distress, anorexia, vomiting, constipation, diarrhea; urinary frequency or retention, dysuria; thickened bronchial secretions, wheezing, chest tightness

Interactions: Alcohol, other CNS depressants, and MAOIs compound CNS depression

5. EPINEPHRINE

Class: Autonomic nervous system agent – natural and synthetic catecholamine; alpha- and beta-adrenergic agonist; bronchodilator

Action: Sympathomimetic that acts directly on both alpha and beta receptors; the most potent activator of alpha receptors; strengthens myocardial contraction; increases systolic but may decrease diastolic blood pressure; increases cardiac rate and output; constricts bronchial arterioles and inhibits histamine release, thus reducing congestion and edema and increasing tidal volume and vital capacity

Dose: 0.1–0.5 mL SC/IM q10–15min (1:1000 soln = 1mg/1ml)

Indications: For hypersensitivity and anaphylactic reactions, acute asthma attack, bronchospasm, mucosal congestion, syncope due to heart block or carotid sinus hypersensitivity, and to restore cardiac rhythm in cardiac arrest; prolong action and delay absorption of anesthetics; control superficial bleeding

Contraindications: Sympathomimetic amine hypersensitivity; narrow-angle glaucoma; hemorrhagic, traumatic, or cardiogenic shock; cardiac dilatation, cerebral arteriosclerosis, coronary insufficiency, arrhythmias, organic heart or brain disease; do NOT use with local anesthesia of fingers, toes, ears, nose, genitalia; pregnancy category C

Adverse Effects: Nervousness, restlessness, sleeplessness, fear, anxiety, tremors, headache, CVA, weakness, dizziness, syncope, pallor, sweating, dyspnea; nausea, vomiting; precordial pain, palpitations, hypertension, MI, tachyarrhythmias; bronchial and pulmonary edema; urinary retention; tissue necrosis; metabolic acidoses; altered state of perception and thought, psychosis

Interactions: May increase hypotension in circulatory collapse; additive toxicities with other medications

6. ERTAPENEM (INVANZ)

Class: Antimicrobial – antibiotic, carbapenem, beta-lactam

Action: Broad-spectrum antibiotic that inhibits cell wall synthesis of gram-positive and gram-negative bacteria by its strong affinity for bacterial cell wall penicillin-binding proteins (PBPs); highly resistant to most bacterial beta-lactamases; effective against most *Enterobacteriaceae, Pseudomonas aeruginosa*, and *Acinetobacter spp;* poorly effective against *Enterococci*, particularly vancomycin-resistant strains

Dose: 1g IV/IM q24h (For IV reconstitute with 10mL NS; for IM 3.2mL 1.0% lidocaine without epinephrine)

Indications: For complicated infections of abdomen, pelvis, urinary tract, and skin; also used for community-acquired pneumonia

Contraindications: Carbapenem, beta-lactam, or amide-type local anesthetic (ie. Lidocaine) hypersensitivity; pregnancy category B

Adverse Effects: Injection site phlebitis or thrombosis; asthenia, fatigue, death, fever, leg pain, anxiety, altered mental status, dizziness, headache, insomnia; chest pain, hypo- or hypertension, tachycardia, edema; abdominal pain, diarrhea, acid reflux, constipation, dyspepsia, nausea, vomiting, increased LFTs; cough, dyspnea, pharyngitis, rales, rhonchi, respiratory distress; erythema, pruritus, rash

Interactions: Probenecid decreases renal excretion

7. FENTANYL ORAL LOZENGES (ACTIQ) - CONTROLLED SUBSTANCE: SCHEDULE II

Class: CNS agent - potent narcotic (opiate) agonist

Action: Action similar to morphine with more rapid and less prolonged analgesia and sedation, but less emetic effect

Dose: 400-800 mcg oral-tranmucosally, titrate to pain up to max 1600 mcg/d; lozenge on a stick to be placed in mouth between cheek and lower gum and sucked, not chewed (have opioid antagonist [naloxone] immediately available!)

Indications: For moderate to severe pain management

Contraindications: MAOIs; myasthenia gravis; pregnancy category C

Side Effects: Sedation, euphoria, dizziness, diaphoresis, delirium, convulsions; bradycardia, hypotension, circulatory depression, cardiac arrest; miosis, blurred vision; nausea, vomiting, constipation, ileus; muscle and thoracic muscle rigidity; urinary retention, rash; laryngospasm, bronchoconstriction, respiratory depression or arrest have

Interactions: Alcohol and other CNS depressants potentiate effects; MAOIs may precipitate hypertensive crisis

8. GATIFLOXACIN (TEQUIN)

Class: Antimicrobial – antibiotic; quinolone

Action: Broad spectrum bactericidal agent that inhibits DNA-gyrase topoisomerase II, an enzyme necessary for bacterial replication, transcription, repair and recombination; effective against methicillin-resistant *Staphylococcus aureus* (MRSA), penicillin resistant *Streptococcus pneumoniae, Pseudomonas aeruginosa,* and cocci resistant to other quinolones

Dose: 400 mg PO/IV daily x 1–14 days (duration dependent on diagnosis)

Indications: For acute bacterial exacerbation of chronic bronchitis; acute sinusitis; community-acquired pneumonia; urinary tract infections; pyelonephritis; gonorrhea

Contraindications: Quinolone hypersensitivity; pregnancy category C

Adverse Effects: Headache, allergic reactions, chills, fever; back pain, chest pain; dizziness, abnormal dreams, insomnia, paresthesia, tremor, vasodilatation, vertigo; palpitation; peripheral edema; nausea, vomiting, diarrhea, abdominal pain, constipation, dyspepsia, glossitis, stomatitis; dyspnea, pharyngitis; rash, sweating; dysuria; hematuria; abnormal vision; taste perversion; tinnitus; increased seizure risk

Interactions: Ferrous sulfate and aluminum or magnesium containing antacids reduce absorption; may cause false positive on opiate screening tests

9. HETASTARCH (HEXTEND)

Class: Plasma volume expander – colloid; synthetic starch resembling human glycogen

Action: Increases colloidal osmotic pressure and expands plasma volume similar to albumin, but with less potential for anaphylaxis or interference with cross matching or blood typing procedures; remains in the intravascular space increasing arterial and venous pressures, heart rate, cardiac output, urine output; not a blood or plasma substitute

Dose: 500–1000 mL IV (max rate: 20 mL/kg/h, max dose: 1500 mL/day); max rate used for acute hemorrhagic shock, reduced rates used with burns or septic shock

Indications: For fluid replacement and plasma volume expansion when blood or plasma is not available, and for adjunctive treatment of shock caused by hemorrhage, burns, surgery, sepsis, or other trauma

Contraindications: Severe bleeding disorders, CHF, renal failure with oliguria and anuria, treatment of shock without hypovolemia, pregnancy category C

Adverse Effects: Peripheral edema, circulatory overload, heart failure; prolonged PT/PTT, clotting time, and bleeding time with large doses; decreased Hb/Hct, platelets, calcium, and fibrinogen; dilution of plasma proteins, hyperbilirubinemia, increased sedimentation rate; pruritus, anaphylactoid reactions (periorbital edema, urticaria, wheezing), vomiting, fever, chills, flu-like symptoms, headache, muscle pains, submaxillary and parotid gland swelling

Interactions: No clinically significant interactions established

---

10. IBUPROFEN (MOTRIN, ADVIL)

Class: CNS agent – NSAID (cox-1); anti-inflammatory, analgesic, antipyretic

Action: Propionic acid inhibitor prototype that blocks prostaglandin synthesis, modulates T-cell function, inhibits inflammatory cell chemotaxis, decreases release of superoxide radicals or increases scavenging of these compounds at inflammatory sites, inhibits platelet aggregation and prolongs bleeding time

Dose: 400–800 mg PO tid-qid (max: 3200 mg/d)

Indications: For mild to moderate pain management, symptomatic relief of arthritis, and to reduce fever

Contraindications: NSAID or aspirin induced urticaria, severe rhinitis, bronchospasm, angioedema, nasal polyps; active peptic ulcer, bleeding abnormalities; pregnancy category B

Adverse Effects: Headache, dizziness, light-headedness, anxiety, emotional lability, fatigue, malaise, drowsiness, anxiety, confusion, depression, aseptic meningitis; hypertension, palpitation, CHF; peripheral edema; amblyopia (blurred vision, decreased visual acuity, scotomas, changes in color vision); nystagmus, visual-field defects; tinnitus, impaired hearing; dry mouth, gingival ulcerations, dyspepsia, heartburn, nausea, vomiting, anorexia, diarrhea, constipation, bloating, flatulence, epigastric or abdominal discomfort or pain, GI ulceration, occult blood loss; thrombocytopenia, neutropenia, hemolytic or aplastic anemia, leukopenia; decreased Hgb/Hct; acute renal failure, polyuria, azotemia, cystitis, hematuria, nephrotoxicity, decreased creatinine clearance; maculopapular and vesicobullous skin eruptions, erythema multiforme, pruritus, acne; fluid retention with edema, Stevens-Johnson syndrome, toxic hepatitis, hypersensitivity reactions, anaphylaxis, bronchospasm, serum sickness, SLE, angioedema

Interactions: Oral anticoagulants and heparin may prolong bleeding time; may increase lithium and methotrexate toxicity; herbals (feverfew, garlic, ginger, ginkgo) may increase risk of bleeding; do not take aspirin concurrently; concurrent alcohol use may increase risk of GI ulceration and bleeding tendencies

11. KETOROLAC (TORADOL)

Class: CNS agent – NSAID; anti-inflammatory, analgesic, antipyretic

Action: Inhibits prostaglandin synthesis

Dose: 15-30 mg IV/IM q6h (max: 150 mg/d on first day, then 120 mg subsequent days); 10 mg PO q6h (max: 40 mg/d); max duration all routes 5 days

Indications: For moderate pain management

Contraindications: Ketorolac hypersensitivity; nasal polyps; angioedema or bronchospastic reaction to aspirin or other NSAIDs; severe renal impairment or renal failure due to volume depletion; patients with risk of bleeding; active peptic ulcer disease; pre- or intraoperatively; pregnancy category B

Adverse Effects: Drowsiness, dizziness, headache; nausea, dyspepsia, GI pain, hemorrhage; edema, sweating

Interactions: May increase methotrexate and lithium levels and toxicity; herbals (feverfew, garlic, ginger, ginkgo) increase bleeding potential

12. LIDOCAINE (XYLOCAINE)

Class: Amide-type local anesthetic; cardiovascular agent; class IB antiarrhythmic

Action: Anesthetic effect similar to procaine; class IB antiarrhythmic action by suppressing automaticity in the His-Purkinje system and by elevating the electrical stimulation threshold of ventricles during diastole

Dose: For local anesthesia, infiltrate 0.5%–2% injection with and without epinephrine

Indications: For surface, infiltration, and nerve block anesthesia; also used for rapid control of ventricular arrhythmias

Contraindications: Amide-type local anesthetic hypersensitivity; systemic injection in presence of severe trauma or sepsis, blood dyscrasias, supraventricular arrhythmias, untreated sinus bradycardia, severe degrees of sinoatrial, atrioventricular, and intraventricular heart block; pregnancy category B

Adverse Effects: Drowsiness, dizziness, light-headedness, restlessness, confusion, disorientation, irritability, apprehension, euphoria, wild excitement, numbness of lips or tongue, hot and cold parasthesia, chest heaviness, difficulty speaking, difficulty breathing or swallowing, muscular twitching, tremors, psychosis; convulsions, respiratory depression and arrest, hypotension, bradycardia, conduction disorders, heart block, cardiovascular collapse, and cardiac arrest in high doses; tinnitus, decreased hearing; blurred or double vision; impaired color perception; local erythema and edema; anorexia, nausea, vomiting; excessive perspiration, thrombophlebitis; urticaria, rash, edema, anaphylactoid reaction

Interactions: Barbiturates decrease activity; cimetidine, beta blockers, quinidine increase effects; phenytoin increases cardiac depressant effects; procainamide compounds neurologic and cardiac effects

13. MELOXICAM (MOBIC)

Class: CNS agent – NSAID; anti-inflammatory, analgesic, antipyretic

Action: Inhibits cyclooxygenase

Dose: 7.5–15 mg PO daily

Indications: For mild to moderate pain management, osteoarthritis, rheumatoid arthritis

Contraindications: NSAID or salicylate hypersensitivity; rhinitis, urticaria, angioedema, asthma; severe renal or hepatic disease; pregnancy category C ($1^{st}/2^{nd}$ trimester) and category D (3rd trimester)

Adverse Effects: Edema, flu-like syndrome, pain; abdominal pain, diarrhea, dyspepsia, flatulence, nausea, constipation, ulceration, GI bleed; anemia; arthralgia; dizziness, headache, insomnia; pharyngitis, upper respiratory tract infection, cough; rash, pruritus; urinary frequency, UTI

Interactions: May decrease effect of ACE inhibitors and diuretics; may increase lithium levels and toxicity; aspirin may increase GI bleed risk; warfarin and herbals (feverfew, garlic, ginger, ginkgo) may increase bleeding

14. MORPHINE SULFATE (MSO4) - CONTROLLED SUBSTANCE: SCHEDULE II

Class: CNS agent – narcotic (opiate) agonist; analgesic

Action: Natural opium alkaloid with agonist activity as it binds with 3 types of the same receptors as endogenous opioid peptides; analgesia at supraspinal level, euphoria, respiratory depression and physical dependence; sedation and miosis; dysphoric, hallucinogenic, and cardiac stimulant effects

Dose: 5–15mg slow IV push, titrate to pain (have opioid antagonist [naloxone] immediately available!)

Indications: For severe acute and chronic pain management, MI pain relief, preanesthesia and as adjunct to anesthesia, and for relief of dyspnea from acute left ventricular failure and pulmonary edema

Contraindications: Opiate hypersensitivity; increased ICP; seizures; acute alcoholism; acute bronchial asthma, chronic pulmonary disease, severe respiratory depression; chemical-irritant induced pulmonary edema; BPH; diarrhea due to poisoning until toxic material has been eliminated; undiagnosed acute abdominal conditions; following biliary tract surgery and surgical anastomosis; pancreatitis; acute ulcerative colitis; severe liver or renal insufficiency; hypothyroidism; pregnancy category B

Adverse Effects: Pruritus, rash, urticaria, edema, anaphylactoid reaction; sweating, skeletal muscle flaccidity; cold, clammy skin, hypothermia; euphoria, insomnia, disorientation, visual disturbances, dysphoria, paradoxic CNS stimulation (restlessness, tremor, delirium, insomnia), convulsions; decreased cough reflex, drowsiness, dizziness, deep sleep, coma; miosis; bradycardia, palpitations, syncope; flushing of face, neck, and upper thorax; orthostatic hypotension, cardiac arrest; constipation, anorexia, dry mouth, biliary colic, nausea, vomiting, elevated LFTs; urinary retention or urgency, dysuria, oliguria, reduced libido or potency; severe respiratory depression or arrest; pulmonary edema

Interactions: CNS depressants, sedatives, barbiturates, alcohol, benzodiazepines, and TCAs potentiate CNS depressant effects; MAOIs may precipitate hypertensive crisis; phenothiazines may antagonize analgesia; herbals (Kava-kava, valerian, St. John's wort) may increase sedation

15. MOXIFLOXACIN (AVELOX)

Class: Antimicrobial – antibiotic; fluoroquinolone

Action: Broad spectrum bactericidal agent that inhibits DNA-gyrase topoisomerase II, an enzyme necessary for bacterial replication, transcription, repair and recombination; effective against gram-positive and gram-negative organisms, *Staphylococcus aureus, Streptococcus pneumonia, Haemophilus influenzae, Klebsiella pneumoniae, Moraxella catarrhalis, Chlamydia pneumoniae, Mycoplasma pneumoniae,* and other microbes

Dose: 400 mg PO/IV daily x 5-10 days

Indications: For acute bacterial exacerbation of chronic bronchitis, acute sinusitis, community-acquired pneumonia, skin infections

Contraindications: Quinolone hypersensitivity; hepatic insufficiency; syphilis; arrhythmias; myocardial ischemia or infarction; QT_c prolongation, hypokalemia, or those receiving Class IA or Class III antiarrhythmic drugs; pregnancy category C

Adverse Effects: Dizziness, headache, peripheral neuropathy, nausea, diarrhea, abdominal pain, vomiting, taste perversion, abnormal LFTs, dyspepsia, tendon rupture

Interactions: Iron, zinc, antacids, aluminum, magnesium, calcium, sucralfate decrease absorption; atenolol, cisapride, erythromycin, antipsychotics, TCAs, quinidine, procainamide, amiodarone, sotalol may prolong QT_c interval; may cause false positive on opiate screening tests

16. NALOXONE (NARCAN)

Class: CNS agent – narcotic (opiate) antagonist

Action: A "pure" narcotic antagonist, essentially free of agonistic (morphine-like) properties; thus, produces no significant analgesia, respiratory depression, psychotomimetic effects, or miosis when administered in the absence of narcotics and possesses more potent narcotic antagonist action

Dose: 0.4–2.0 mg IV, repeat q2–3min up to 10 mg prn

Indications: For narcotic opiate overdose and reversal of effects of natural and synthetic narctotics (opiates), including respiratory depression, sedation, and hypotension; drug of choice when depressant drug is unknown and for diagnosis of suspected acute opioid overdose

Contraindications: Non-opioid drug respiratory depression; pregnancy category B

Adverse Effects: Analgesia reversal, tremors, hyperventilation, drowsiness, sweating; increased BP, tachycardia; nausea, vomiting; elevated PTT

Interactions: Reverses analgesic effects of narcotic (opiate) agonists and agonist-antagonists

17. PROMETHAZINE (PHENERGAN)

Class: GI agent – phenothiazine; antiemetic, antivertigo

Action: Long-acting phenothiazine derivative with prominent sedative, amnesic, antiemetic, and anti-motion-sickness actions and marked antihistamine activity; antiemetic action due to depression of CTZ in medulla; as with other antihistamines, it exerts antiserotonin, anticholinergic, and local anesthetic action

Dose: 12.5-25 mg PO/IM/IV q4-6h prn

Indications: For symptomatic relief from nausea, vomiting, motion sickness, and allergic conditions; also used for pre- and postoperative sedation, and as adjunct to analgesics for control of pain

Contraindications: Phenothiazine hypersensitivity; narrow-angle glaucoma; stenosing peptic ulcer, pyloroduodenal obstruction; BPH; bladder neck obstruction; epilepsy; bone marrow depression; comatose or severe depressed states; Reye's syndrome, encephalopathy, hepatic diseases; pregnancy category C

Adverse Effects: Deep sleep, coma, convulsions, cardiorespiratory symptoms, extrapyramidal reactions, nightmares, CNS stimulation, abnormal movements; irregular respirations, respiratory depression; sedation drowsiness, confusion, dizziness, disturbed coordination, restlessness, tremors; transient mild hypo- or hypertension; anorexia, nausea, vomiting, constipation; leukopenia, agranulocytosis; blurred vision, dry mouth, nose, or throat; photosensitivity; urinary retention

Interactions: Alcohol and other CNS depressants add to CNS depression and anticholinergic effects

18. SODIUM CHLORIDE, 0.9% (NORMAL SALINE)

Class: Plasma volume expander – crystalloid; isotonic salt solution

Action: Each mL contains 9 g sodium chloride (Na+ 154 mEq/L; Cl⁻ 154 mEq/L); pH 5.7; expands circulating volume by approximating sodium content of the blood; but, it remains in the intravascular space for only a very limited time as it diffuses rapidly throughout the extracellular space

Dose: 500–1000 mL IV; 5-50 mL IV for medication dilution or as flush

Indications: For fluid replacement and plasma volume expansion when blood or plasma is not available, and for adjunctive treatment of shock and hypovolemic states caused by hemorrhage, burns, surgery, sepsis, trauma, dehydration, or heat injury; also used for dilution of medications, as IV flush agent, for saline locks, and irrigation of eyes and wounds

Contraindications: CHF

Adverse Effects: Fluid overload, CHF, edema, electrolyte imbalance, hyperchloremic metabolic acidosis, hypertension

Interactions: No clinically significant interactions established

SECTION THREE

RMED
PHARMACOLOGY
SECTION II

"PROFICIENT"

PHARMACOLOGY SECTION II: "PROFICIENT"

1. ACETAZOLAMIDE (DIAMOX)   250 mg PO q8–12h from 1-2 d prior, to ≥ 5d at alt.
2. ACETYLSALICYLIC ACID (ASPIRIN)   325–650 mg PO/PR q4h
3. ALBUTEROL (PROVENTIL)   MDI 2 puffs q4–6h prn
4. BACITRACIN   Topical ointment to AAA bid-tid
5. BENZONATATE (TESSALON PERLES)   100-200 mg PO tid prn (max 600 mg/d)
6. CEFTRIAXONE (ROCEPHIN)   1–2 g IV/IM q12–24h (max: 4 g/d)
7. CETIRIZINE (ZYRTEC)   5–10mg PO qd
8. CIMETIDINE (TAGAMET)   300 mg IV/IM/PO q6-8h or 400 mg po bid
9. CLINDAMYCIN (CLEOCIN)   150–450 mg PO q6h; 600–900 mg IM/IV q6–8h
10. DEXTROMETHORPHAN (ROBITUSSIN DM)   10–20 mg PO q4h or 30 mg q6–8h (max: 120 mg/d)
11. DEXTROSE (D50)   0.5-1 g/kg (1-2 ml/kg) up to 25 g (50 mL) IV
12. DOXYCYCLINE   100 mg PO qd from 1-2 d prior to 4 wks after expos
13. FEXOFENADINE (ALLEGRA)   60 mg PO bid or 180 mg PO qd
14. GUAIFENESIN   100–400 mg PO q4h or 600-1200 mg XR PO q12h
15. HYDROCORTISONE   topically AAA qd-qid
16. HYDROMORPHONE (DILAUDID)   1–4 mg PO/SC/IM/IV q4–6h prn
17. LACTATED RINGER'S (LR)   500-1000 mL IV
18. LEVOFLOXACIN (LEVAQUIN)   250-750 mg PO/IV daily
19. LOPERAMIDE (IMODIUM)   4 mg PO, then 2 mg with loose BM (max: 16 mg/d)
20. LORATADINE (CLARITIN)   10 mg PO daily
21. MECLIZINE (ANTIVERT)   25–50 mg PO 1 h before travel
22. MEFLOQUINE (LARIUM)   250 mg PO once/wk from 1 wk prior to 4 wks after
23. ONDANSETRON (ZOFRAN)   8-16 mg PO q8h prn; 4mg slow IVP or IM q8h prn
24. PRIMAQUINE   30 mg base PO daily x 14 d, after malaria exposure
25. PSEUDOEPHEDRINE (SUDAFED)   30-60 mg PO q4–6h or 120 mg XR PO q12h
26. RANITIDINE (ZANTAC)   75-150 mg PO bid or 150-300 mg PO qhs
27. TMP-SMZ (BACTRIM, SEPTRA)   160 mg TMP/800 mg SMZ (DS) PO bid
28. ZOLPIDEM (AMBIEN)   5–10 mg PO qhs, limited to 7–10 days

1. ACETAZOLAMIDE (DIAMOX)

Class: CNS Agent – carbonic anhydrase inhibitor; diuretic, anticonvulsant

Action: Diuretic effect due to inhibition of carbonic anhydrase activity in proximal renal tubule, preventing formation of carbonic acid; anticonvulsant action effect thought to involve inhibition of CNS carbonic anhydrase, retarding abnormal paroxysmal discharge from CNS neurons

Dose: 250 mg PO q8–12h; 500 mg SR q12–24h; start 1-2 d prior, continue for ≥ 5 d while at high altitude

Indications: For acute high-altitude sickness, seizures, drug-induced edema, and for CHF edema

Contraindications: Sulfonamide and thiazide hypersensitivity; marked renal and hepatic dysfunction; adrenocortical insufficiency; hyponatremia, hypokalemia, hyperchloremic acidosis; pregnancy category C

Adverse Effects: Paresthesias, sedation, malaise, disorientation, depression, fatigue, muscle weakness, flaccid paralysis; anorexia, nausea, vomiting, weight loss, dry mouth, thirst, diarrhea; agranulocytosis, bone marrow depression, hemolytic anemia, aplastic anemia, leukopenia, pancytopenia; hyperglycemia; hyperuricemia; increased calcium, potassium, magnesium, sodium excretion; gout exacerbation, dysuria, glycosuria, urinary frequency, polyuria, hematuria, crystalluria; metabolic acidosis; hepatic dysfunction

Interactions: Renal excretion of amphetamines, ephedrine, flecainide, quinidine, procainamide, TCAs may be decreased, thereby enhancing or prolonging their effects; renal excretion of lithium and phenobarbital is increased; amphotericin B and corticosteroids may accelerate potassium loss; increased risk for salicylate and digitalis toxicity

2. ACETYLSALICYLIC ACID (ASPIRIN)

Class: CNS agent – NSAID; salicylate; anti-inflammatory, analgesic, antipyretic

Action: Inhibits prostaglandin synthesis involved in the production of inflammation, pain, and fever; enhances antigen removal and reduces spread of inflammation; peripheral analgesic action with limited CNS action in the hypothalamus; antipyretic by indirect centrally mediated peripheral vasodilation and sweating; powerfully inhibits platelet aggregation and ability of blood to clot; high levels can impair hepatic synthesis of blood coagulation factors VII, IX, and X, possibly by inhibiting action of vitamin K

Dose: 325-650 mg PO/PR q4-6h (max: 4 g/d); MI prophylaxis PO 80-325 mg/d (chewable or coated)

Indications: For mild to moderate pain management, fever reduction, and to decrease inflammation; also used for acute rheumatic fever, Systemic Lupus, rheumatoid arthritis, osteoarthritis, bursitis, calcific tendonitis, to reduce recurrence of TIA and risk of stroke, as prophylaxis and to prevent recurrence of MI

Contraindications: Salicylate and NSAID hypersensitivity; patients with "aspirin triad" (aspirin sensitivity, nasal polyps, asthma); chronic rhinitis or urticaria; GI ulcer, bleeding; hypoprothrombinemia, vitamin K deficiency, hemophilia, bleeding disorders; CHF; pregnancy category D; do NOT use in children or teenagers with viral illnesses due to link with Reye's syndrome

Adverse Effects: Rash, urticaria, easy bruising, petechiae, bronchospasm, laryngeal edema; confusion, dizziness, drowsiness; tinnitus, hearing loss; nausea, vomiting, diarrhea, anorexia, heartburn, stomach pain, GI bleeding, ulceration; thrombocytopenia, hemolytic anemia, prolonged bleeding time

Interactions: Aminosalicylic acid and carbonic anhydrase inhibitors increase risk of toxicity; ammonium chloride, acidifying agents decrease renal elimination and increase toxicity; oral hypoglycemic agents increase hypoglycemic activity; corticosteroids increase ulcer potential; methotrexate toxicity is increased; anticoagulants and herbals (feverfew, garlic, ginger, ginkgo) increase bleeding potential

3. ALBUTEROL (PROVENTIL)

Class: Autonomic nervous system agent – sympathomimetic, beta-adrenergic agonist, bronchodilator

Action: Acts more prominently on beta$_2$ receptors (particularly smooth muscles of bronchi, uterus, and vascular supply to skeletal muscles) than on beta$_1$ (heart) receptors; minimal or no effect on alpha-adrenergic receptors; inhibits histamine release by mast cells; produces bronchodilation, by relaxing smooth muscles of bronchial tree which decreases airway resistance, facilitates mucus drainage, and increases vital capacity

Dose: MDI 2 puffs q4–6h prn; NEB 0.5 mL of 0.5% soln (2.5 mg) in 5 mL NS nebulized tid-qid

Indications: For prevention of exercise-induced bronchospasm, or relief of bronchospasm associated with acute or chronic asthma, bronchitis, or other reversible obstructive airway disease; also used 20–30 minutes before inhaled steroids to allow for deeper penetration of the steroids into the lungs

Contraindications: Pregnancy category C

Adverse Effects: Hypersensitivity reaction, tremor, anxiety, nervousness, restlessness, convulsions, weakness, headache, hallucinations; palpitation, hyper- or hypotension, bradycardia, reflex tachycardia; blurred vision, dilated pupils; nausea, vomiting; muscle cramps, hoarseness

Interactions: Additive effect with epinephrine and other sympathomimetic bronchodilators; MAOIs and TCAs potentiate action on vascular system; beta-adrenergic blockers antagonize effects

4. BACITRACIN

Class: Antimicrobial – antibiotic

Action: Polypeptide derived from *Bacillus subtilis* culture; bactericidal/bacteriostatic that appears to inhibit cell wall synthesis; activity similar to penicillin; active against many gram-positives including *Streptococci, Staphylococci, Pneumococci, Corynebacteria, Clostridia, Neisseria, Gonococci, Meningococci, Haemophilus influenzae,* and *Treponema pallidum*; ineffective against most other gram-negatives

Dose: Topical ointment to AAA bid-tid, clean affected area prior to application

Indications: For topical treatment of superficial skin infections

Contraindications: Atopic individuals; pregnancy category C

Adverse Effects: Bacitracin hypersensitivity (erythema, anaphylaxis)

Interactions: No clinically significant interactions established when given topically

5. BENZONATATE (TESSALON PERLES)

Class: ENT agent – antitussive

Action: Nonnarcotic antitussive chemically related to tetracaine; does not inhibit respiratory center at recommended doses; decreases frequency and intensity of nonproductive cough

Dose: 100-200 mg PO tid prn (max 600 mg/d)

Indications: For management of nonproductive cough in acute and chronic respiratory conditions

Contraindications: Pregnancy category C

Adverse Effects: Drowsiness, sedation, headache, mild dizziness; constipation, nausea; rash, pruritus

Interactions: Swallow whole; do not chew or dissolve as mouth, tongue, pharynx will be anesthetized

6. CEFTRIAXONE (ROCEPHIN)

Class: Antimicrobial – antibiotic; third-generation cephalosporin

Action: Preferentially binds to penicillin-binding proteins (PBP) and inhibits bacterial cell wall synthesis; effective against most *Enterobacteriaceae,* gram-positive aerobic cocci, *Neisseria meningitides and gonorrhoeae*; some effect against *Treponema pallidum*

Dose: For moderate to severe infections, 1–2 g IV/IM q12–24h (max: 4 g/d); for meningitis, 2 g IV/IM q12h; for uncomplicated gonorrhea 250 mg IM x 1; dilute in 1% lidocaine for IM

Indications: For infections of the middle ear, lower respiratory tract, skin and skin structures, bones and joints, meningitis, intra-abdominal, urogenital tract, pelvis, septicemia; used for surgical prophylaxis

Contraindications: Cephalosporin hypersensitivity; pregnancy category B

Adverse Effects: Pruritus, fever, chills, pain, induration at IM site; phlebitis at IV site; diarrhea, abdominal cramps, pseudomembranous colitis, biliary sludge

Interactions: Probenecid decreases renal elimination; alcohol produces disulfiram reaction

7. CETIRIZINE (ZYRTEC)

Class: ENT agent – H_1-receptor antagonist; non-sedating antihistamine

Action: Potent H_1-receptor antagonist and antihistamine; low lipophilicity and H_1-receptor selectivity and thus no significant anticholinergic or CNS activity; reduces local and systemic effects of histamine release

Dose: 5–10mg PO qd

Indications: Seasonal and perennial allergic rhinitis and chronic idiopathic urticaria

Contraindications: H_1-receptor antihistamine hypersensitivity; pregnancy category B

Adverse Effects: Constipation, diarrhea, dry mouth; drowsiness, sedation, headache, depression

Interactions: Theophylline may decrease clearance leading to toxicity; do not use in combination with OTC antihistamines

8. CIMETIDINE (TAGAMET)

Class: GI agent – antisecretory H2-receptor antagonist

Action: Antihistamine with high selectivity for reversible competitive inhibition of histamine H_2-receptors on parietal cells of the stomach (minimal effect on H_1-receptors) and thus decreases gastric acid secretion, raises the pH of the stomach, and indirectly reduces pepsin secretion

Dose: 300 mg IV/IM/PO q6-8h or 400 mg po bid or 400-800 mg qhs

Indications: For treatment of duodenal/gastric ulcer, prevention of ulcer recurrence, gastroesophageal reflux, chronic urticaria, acetaminophen toxicity

Contraindications: H_2 receptor antagonists hypersensitivity; pregnancy category B

Adverse Effects: Fever; cardiac arrhythmias and cardiac arrest after rapid IV bolus; diarrhea, constipation, abdominal discomfort; increased prothrombin time; neutropenia, thrombocytopenia, aplastic anemia; hypospermia; exacerbation of preexisting arthritis; drowsiness, dizziness, light-headedness, depression, headache, reversible confusional states, paranoid psychosis; rash, Stevens-Johnson syndrome, reversible alopecia; gynecomastia, galactorrhea, reversible impotence

Interactions: Decreases hepatic metabolism of warfarin, phenobarbital, phenytoin, diazepam, propranolol, lidocaine, theophylline, thus increasing their activity and toxicity; antacids may decrease absorption

9. CLINDAMYCIN (CLEOCIN)

Class: Antimicrobial – antibiotic

Action: Suppresses protein synthesis by binding to 50 S subunits of bacterial ribosomes; effective against strains of anaerobic streptococci, *Bacteroides* (especially *B. fragilis*), *Fusobacterium, Actinomyces israelii, Peptococcus, Clostridium sp*, and aerobic gram-positive cocci, including *Staphylococcus aureus, Staphylococcus epidermidis, Streptococci* (except *S. faecalis*), and *Pneumococci*

Dose: Cleocin: 150–450 mg PO q6h; 600–900 mg IM/IV q6–8h (max: 2700 mg/d), each IM injection ≤ 600 mg; Cleocin T: topically AAA BID

Indications: For moderate to severe infections; topical applications used in treatment of acne vulgaris

Contraindications: Clindamycin or lincomycin hypersensitivity; history of regional enteritis, ulcerative colitis, or antibiotic-associated colitis; pregnancy category B

Adverse Effects: Fever, serum sickness, sensitization, swelling of face, generalized myalgia, superinfections, proctitis, pain, induration, sterile abscess; thrombophlebitis; hypotension, cardiac arrest (rapid IV); diarrhea, abdominal pain, flatulence, bloating, nausea, vomiting, pseudomembranous colitis; esophageal irritation, loss of taste, medicinal taste (high IV doses), jaundice, abnormal liver function tests; leukopenia, eosinophilia, agranulocytosis, thrombocytopenia; skin rashes, urticaria, pruritus, dryness, contact dermatitis, gram-negative folliculitis, irritation, oily skin

Interactions: Chloramphenicol and erythromycin are possibly antagonistic; neuromuscular blocking action enhanced by neuromuscular blocking agents (atracurium, tubocurarine, pancuronium)

10. DEXTROMETHORPHAN (ROBITUSSIN DM)

Class: ENT agent – Antitussive

Action: Nonnarcotic derivative that depresses the cough center in the medulla; chemically related to morphine but without central hypnotic or analgesic effect or capacity to cause tolerance or addiction; antitussive activity comparable to that of codeine but is less likely than codeine to cause constipation, drowsiness, or GI disturbance

Dose: 10–20 mg PO q4h or 30 mg q6–8h (max: 120 mg/d)

Indication: For temporary relief or control of cough spasms in nonproductive coughs due to colds, pertussis, or influenza

Contraindications: Asthma; productive or persistent cough; liver impairment; pregnancy category C

Adverse Effects: Dizziness, drowsiness, CNS depression with very large doses; excitability; GI upset, constipation, abdominal discomfort

Interactions: MAOIs can cause excitation, hypotension, and hyperpyrexia; CNS depressants can cause dizziness and drowsiness

11. DEXTROSE (D50)

Class: Endocrine agent – caloric, monosaccharide

Action: Needed for adequate utilization of amino acids, decreases protein and nitrogen loss, and prevents ketosis

Dose: 0.5-1 g/kg (1-2 ml/kg) up to 25 g (50 mL) of 50% solution IV; if tolerating PO, provide glucose tabs

Indication: For treatment of hypoglycemic episode

Contraindications: Hyperglycemia, delirium tremens, cranial or spinal hemorrhage, CHF

Adverse Effects: Confusion, loss of consciousness, dizziness; hypertension, CHF, pulmonary edema; glycosuria, osmotic diuresis; hyperglycemia, rebound hypoglycemia; chills, flushing, rash, urticaria

Interactions: No clinically significant interactions established

12. DOXYCYCLINE

Class: Antimicrobial – antibiotic; tetracycline

Action: Semisynthetic broad-spectrum antibiotic derived from oxytetracycline, but more completely absorbed with effective blood levels maintained for longer periods and excreted more slowly than most other tetracyclines, thus it requires smaller and less frequent dosing; primarily bacteriostatic in effect

Dose: As antimalarial, 100 mg PO qd starting 1-2 days prior to 4 wks after exposure; as antimicrobial, 100 mg PO q12h on day 1, then 100 mg qd; for travelers' diarrhea, 100 PO QD during risk period; for gonorrhea, 200 mg PO immediately, followed by 100 mg bid x 3 d; for syphilis 100 mg PO tid x 10 d; for acne, 100 mg PO qd-bid

Indications: For suppression and chemoprophylaxis of chloroquine-resistant *Plasmodium falciparum* malaria, short-term prophylaxis and treatment of travelers' diarrhea caused by enterotoxigenic strains of *Escherichia coli*, Chlamydial and mycoplasmal infections, gonorrhea, syphilis in penicillin-allergic patients, rickettsial diseases, acute exacerbations of chronic bronchitis, and treatment of acne

Contraindications: Tetracycline hypersensitivity; use during period of tooth development including last half of pregnancy causes permanent yellow discoloration of teeth, enamel hypoplasia, and retardation of bone growth, pregnancy category D

Adverse Effects: Interference with color vision; anorexia, nausea, vomiting, diarrhea, enterocolitis; esophageal irritation; rashes, photosensitivity reaction; superinfections

Interactions: Antacids, iron preparation, calcium, magnesium, zinc, kaolin-pectin, sodium bicarbonate can significantly decrease absorption; effects of both doxycycline and desmopressin antagonized; increases digoxin absorption and risk of toxicity; methoxyflurane increases risk of renal failure

13. FEXOFENADINE (ALLEGRA)

Class: ENT agent – H_1-receptor antagonist; non-sedating antihistamine

Action: Competitively antagonizes histamine at the H_1-receptor site; does not bind with histamine to inactivate it; not associated with anticholinergic or sedative properties; inhibits antigen-induced bronchospasm and histamine release from mast cells

Dose: 60 mg PO bid or 180 mg PO qd

Indications: For symptom relief from seasonal allergic rhinitis (nasal congestion and sneezing; watery or red eyes; itching nose, palate, or eyes) and chronic urticaria

Contraindications: Fexofenadine hypersensitivity; pregnancy category C

Adverse Effects: Headache, drowsiness, fatigue; nausea, dyspepsia, throat irritation

Interactions: No clinically significant interactions established

14. GUAIFENESIN

Class: ENT agent – antitussive, expectorant

Action: Enhances reflex outflow of respiratory tract fluids by irritation of gastric mucosa; aids in expectoration by reducing adhesiveness and surface tension of secretions

Dose: 100–400 mg PO q4h or 600-1200 mg XR PO q12h (max: 2.4 g/d)

Indications: Relief of dry, nonproductive coughs associated with colds and bronchitis

Contraindications: Guaifenesin hypersensitivity; pregnancy category C

Adverse Effects: Low incidence of nausea; drowsiness

Interactions: By inhibiting platelet function, may increase risk of bleeding in patients receiving heparin

15. HYDROCORTISONE

Class: Skin and mucous membrane agent – synthetic hormone; adrenal corticosteroid, glucocorticoid, mineralocorticoid, antiinflammatory

Action: Stabilizes leukocyte lysosomal membranes, inhibits phagocytosis and release of allergic substances, suppresses fibroblast formation and collagen deposition

Dose: Topically AAA qd-qid

Indications: To reduce inflammation in various skin conditions

Contraindications: Steroid hypersensitivity, viral or bacterial diseases of skin; varicella or vaccinia on surfaces with compromised circulation; pregnancy category C

Adverse Effects: Anaphylactoid reaction; aggravation or masking of infections; skin thinning and atrophy, acne, impaired wound healing; petechiae, ecchymosis, easy bruising; hypopigmentation or hyperpigmentation, hirsutism, acneiform eruptions, subcutaneous fat atrophy; allergic dermatitis, urticaria, angioneurotic edema, increased sweating

Interactions: Estrogens potentiate effects; immune response to vaccines may be decreased

16. HYDROMORPHONE (DILAUDID) - CONTROLLED SUBSTANCE: SCHEDULE II

Class: CNS agent – narcotic (opiate) agonist; analgesic

Action: Semisynthetic derivative structurally similar to morphine with 8–10 times more potent analgesic effect, more rapid onset, shorter duration of action, less hypnotic effect, and less tendency to produce nausea and vomiting; also has antitussive properties

Dose: 1–4 mg PO/SC/IM/IV q4–6h prn

Indications: For moderate to severe pain management, and control of persistent nonproductive cough

Contraindications: Opiate hypersensitivity; acute bronchial asthma, COPD, decreased respiratory reserve, severe respiratory depression, opiate-naïve patients; pregnancy category C

Adverse Effects: Nausea, vomiting, constipation; euphoria, dizziness, sedation, drowsiness; hypotension, bradycardia, tachycardia; respiratory depression; blurred vision

Interactions: Alcohol and other CNS depressants compound sedation and CNS depression; herbal (St. John's wort) may increase sedation

17. LACTATED RINGER'S (LR)

Class: Plasma volume expander – crystalloid; isotonic salt solution

Action: Each liter contains 6.0 g Sodium Chloride (Na+ 130 mEq/L, Cl⁻ 109 mEq/L) and other electrolytes (K+ 4 mEq/L, Ca++ 3 mEq/L, Lactate 28 mEq/L, and 9 kcal/L); pH 6.4; remains in the intravascular space for only a very limited time as it diffuses rapidly throughout the extracellular space

Dose: 500–1000 mL IV

Indications: For fluid replacement and plasma volume expansion when blood or plasma is not available, and for adjunctive treatment of shock and hypovolemic states caused by hemorrhage, burns, surgery, sepsis, trauma, dehydration, or illness; also used for irrigation

Contraindications: CHF; do not use with blood or blood products

Adverse Effects: Fluid overload, CHF, edema, electrolyte imbalance, hypertension

Interactions: Calcium in LR can bind to other drugs and reduce efficacy, also has potential for creating emboli if given with blood or blood products

18. LEVOFLOXACIN (LEVAQUIN)

Class: Antimicrobial – antibiotic; fluoroquinolone

Action: Broad-spectrum antibiotic that inhibits DNA bacterial topoisomerase II, an enzyme required for DNA replication, transcription, repair, and recombination; prevents replication of certain bacteria resistant to beta-lactam antibiotics

Dose: 250-750 mg PO/IV daily; for community-acquired pneumonia: 750 mg PO qd x 5 d; for chronic bacterial prostatitis: 500 mg PO qd x 28 d; for skin infections: 750 mg PO qd x 14 d

Indications: For treatment of maxillary sinusitis, acute exacerbations of bacterial bronchitis, community-acquired pneumonia, uncomplicated skin/skin structure infections, UTI, acute pyelonephritis; chronic bacterial prostatitis; bacterial conjunctivitis

Contraindications: Quinolone hypersensitivity; hypokalemia; tendon pain; syphilis; viral infections; phototoxicity; pregnancy category C

Adverse Effects: Headache, insomnia, dizziness; nausea, diarrhea, constipation, vomiting, abdominal pain, dyspepsia; rash, pruritus; decreased vision, foreign body sensation, transient ocular burning, ocular pain, photophobia; chest or back pain, fever, pharyngitis.

Interactions: Magnesium or aluminum-containing antacids, sucralfate, iron, and zinc may decrease absorption; NSAIDs may increase risk of CNS reactions including seizures; may cause hyper- or hypoglycemia in patients on oral hypoglycemic agents; may cause false positive on opiate screening tests; avoid exposure to excess sunlight or artificial UV light; avoid NSAIDs while taking levofloxacin

19. LOPERAMIDE (IMODIUM)

Class: GI agent – antidiarrheal

Action: Synthetic piperidine derivative that inhibits GI peristaltic activity by direct action on circular and longitudinal intestinal muscles; prolongs intestinal content transit time, increases consistency of stools, and reduces fluid and electrolyte loss

Dose: 4 mg PO, followed by 2 mg after each unformed stool (max: 16 mg/d)

Indications: For acute nonspecific diarrhea, chronic diarrhea associated with inflammatory bowel disease

Contraindications: Conditions in which constipation should be avoided, severe colitis, acute diarrhea caused by broad-spectrum antibiotics (pseudomembranous colitis) or from organisms that penetrate the intestinal mucosa (toxigenic *Escherichia coli, Salmonella,* or *Shigella*); pregnancy category B

Adverse Effects: Rash; fever; drowsiness, fatigue, dizziness, CNS depression with overdose; abdominal distension, discomfort or pain, bloating, constipation, nausea, vomiting, anorexia, dry mouth; toxic megacolon in patients with ulcerative colitis

Interactions: No clinically significant interactions established

20. LORATADINE (CLARITIN)

Class: ENT agent – H_1-receptor antagonist – non-sedating antihistamine

Action: Long-acting histamine antagonist with selective peripheral H_1-receptor sites that blocks histamine release; disrupts capillary permeability, edema formation, and constriction of respiratory, GI, and vascular smooth muscle

Dose: 10 mg PO daily, take on an empty stomach

Indications: Symptom relief from seasonal allergic rhinitis; idiopathic chronic urticaria

Contraindications: Loratadine hypersensitivity; pregnancy category B

Adverse Effects: Dizziness, dry mouth, fatigue, headache, somnolence, altered salivation and lacrimation, thirst, flushing, anxiety, depression, impaired concentration; hypo- or hypertension, palpitations, syncope, tachycardia; nausea, vomiting, flatulence, abdominal distress, constipation, diarrhea, weight gain, dyspepsia; arthralgia, myalgia; blurred vision, earache, eye pain, tinnitus; rash, pruritus, photosensitivity

Interactions: No clinically significant interactions established

21. MECLIZINE (ANTIVERT)

Class: H1-Receptor antagonist; antihistamine, anti-vertigo agent

Action: Long-acting piperazine antihistamine with marked effect in blocking histamine-induced vasopressive response, but only slight anticholinergic action; marked depressant action on labyrinthine excitability and on conduction in vestibular-cerebellar pathways; exhibits CNS depression, antispasmodic, antiemetic, and local anesthetic activity

Dose: For motion sickness, 25–50 mg PO 1 h before travel, may repeat q24h prn for duration of journey; for vertigo, 25–100 mg/d PO in divided doses

Indications: For management of nausea, vomiting, and dizziness associated with motion sickness and vertigo associated with diseases affecting the vestibular system

Contraindications: Hypersensitivity to meclizine; pregnancy category B

Adverse Effects: Drowsiness; dry mouth; blurred vision; fatigue

Interactions: Alcohol and CNS depressants may potentiate sedative effects; do not drive or engage in potentially hazardous activities until response to drug is known

22. MEFLOQUINE (LARIUM)

Class: Antimicrobial – antimalarial

Action: Antimalarial agent structurally related to quinine; effective against all types of malaria including chloroquine resistant malaria

Dose: For malaria prophylaxis, 250 mg PO once/wk (beginning 1 wk before travel and ending 4 wks after leaving endemic area; for malaria treatment, 1250 mg (5 tablets) PO x 1 single dose

Indications: For prevention of chloroquine-resistant malaria caused by *Plasmodium falciparum* and *P. vivax*, and treatment of mild to moderate acute malarial infections

Contraindications: Mefloquine hypersensitivity; calcium channel blockers, severe heart arrhythmias, history of QTc prolongation; aggressive behavior; active or history of depression or suicidal ideation; anxiety disorder, psychosis, schizophrenia, or other major psychiatric disorder; seizure disorder; pregnancy category C

Adverse Effects: Arthralgia, chills, fatigue, fever; dizziness, nightmares, visual disturbances, headache, syncope, confusion, psychosis, aggression, suicide ideation; bradycardia, ECG changes to include QTc prolongation, first-degree AV block; nausea, vomiting, abdominal pain, anorexia, diarrhea; rash, itching

Interactions: Can prolong cardiac conduction in patients taking beta blockers, calcium channel blockers, and possibly digoxin; quinine may decrease plasma levels; may decrease valproic acid levels by increasing hepatic metabolism; administration with chloroquine may increase risk of seizures; increased risk of cardiac arrest and seizures with quinidine; do not give concurrently with quinine or quinidine

23. ONDANSETRON (ZOFRAN)

Class: GI agent – 5-HT$_3$ antagonist, antiemetic

Action: Selective serotonin (5-HT$_3$) receptor antagonist, acting centrally in the chemoreceptor trigger zone (CTZ) and peripherally on the vagal nerve terminals; serotonin is released from the wall of the small intestine, stimulates the vagal efferents through the serotonin receptors, and initiates the vomiting reflex

Dose: 8-16 mg PO q8h prn; 4mg slow IVP or IM q8h prn

Indications: Prevention of nausea and vomiting associated with anesthesia, postoperative state, and chemotherapy

Contraindications: Hypersensitivity to ondansetron; pregnancy category B

Adverse Effects: Dizziness, light-headedness, headache, sedation; diarrhea, constipation, dry mouth

Interactions: Rifampin may decrease ondansetron levels

24. PRIMAQUINE

Class: Antimicrobial – antimalarial

Action: Acts on primary exoerythrocytic forms of *Plasmodium vivax* and *Plasmodium falciparum* by an incompletely known mechanism. Destroys late tissue forms of *P. vivax* and thus effects radical cure (prevents relapse).

Dose: 30 mg base PO daily x 14 d beginning immediately after leaving malarious area; screen for G6PD deficiency prior to providing; give with meal or with antacid to prevent or relieve gastric irritation

Indication: For gametocidal activity against all species of plasmodia that infect man; interrupts transmission of malaria; used to prevent relapse of *P. vivax* and *P. ovale* malarias and to prevent attacks after departure from areas where *P. vivax* and *P. ovale* malarias are endemic

Contraindications: G6PD deficiency; rheumatoid arthritis; SLE; hemolytic drugs, bone marrow depression; quinacrine; NADH methemoglobin reductase deficiency; pregnancy category C

Adverse Effects: Hematologic reactions to include acute hemolytic anemia if G6PD deficient (an inherited error of metabolism carried on the X chromosome, present in about 10% of American black males and certain ethnic groups: Sardinians, Sephardic Jews, Greeks, and Iranians; whites manifest more intense hemolytic reaction); early hemolytic reaction symptoms include darkening of urine, red-tinged urine, decrease in urine volume, chills, fever, precordial pain, cyanosis; leukocytosis, leukopenia, anemia, granulocytopenia, agranulocytosis; nausea, vomiting, epigastric distress, abdominal cramps; pruritus; methemoglobinemia (cyanosis); headache, confusion, mental depression; visual accommodation disturbances; hypertension, arrhythmias

Interactions: Increased toxicity of both quinacrine and primaquine

25. PSEUDOEPHEDRINE (SUDAFED)

Class: Autonomic nervous system agent–sympathomimetic; alpha/beta-adrenergic agonist, decongestant

Action: Sympathomimetic amine that, like ephedrine, produces decongestion of respiratory tract mucosa by stimulating the sympathetic nerve endings including alpha-, beta-1 and beta-2 receptors; unlike ephedrine, also acts directly on smooth muscle and constricts renal and vertebral arteries; has fewer adverse effects, less pressor action, and longer duration of effects than ephedrine

Dose: 30-60 mg PO q4–6h or 120 mg XR PO q12h

Indications: Symptomatic relief of nasal and eustachian tube congestion, rhinitis, and sinusitis

Contraindications: Sympathomimetic amine hypersensitivity; severe hypertension; coronary artery disease; MAOIs; glaucoma; hyperthyroidism; BPH; pregnancy category C

Adverse Effects: Stimulation, tremulousness, difficulty voiding; arrhythmias, palpitation, tachycardia; nervousness, dizziness, headache, sleeplessness, numbness; anorexia, dry mouth, nausea, vomiting

Interactions: Sympathomimetics and beta blockers increase pressor effects and toxicity; MAOIs may precipitate hypertensive crisis; decreases antihypertensive effects of guanethidine, methyldopa, reserpine

26. RANITIDINE (ZANTAC)

Class: GI agent – antisecretory H2-receptor antagonist

Action: Antihistamine with high selectivity for reversible competitive inhibition of histamine H_2-receptors on parietal cells of the stomach (minimal effect on H_1-receptors) and thus decreases gastric acid secretion, raises the pH of the stomach, and indirectly reduces pepsin secretion

Dose: 75-150 mg PO bid or 150-300 mg PO qhs; 50 mg IV/IM q6–8h

Indications: For treatment of duodenal/gastric ulcers and gastroesophageal reflux disease

Contraindications: Ranitidine hypersensitivity; acute porphyria; pregnancy category B

Adverse Effects: Headache, malaise, dizziness, somnolence, insomnia, vertigo, mental confusion, agitation, depression, hallucinations in older adults; bradycardia (with rapid IV push); constipation, nausea, abdominal pain, diarrhea; rash; reversible decrease in WBC count, thrombocytopenia

Interactions: May reduce absorption of cefpodoxime, cefuroxime, delavirdine, ketoconazole, itraconazole; long-term therapy may lead to vitamin B_{12} deficiency

27. TRIMETHOPRIM-SULFAMETHOXAZOLE (TMP-SMZ, BACTRIM, SEPTRA)

Class: Antimicrobial – antibacterial, sulfonamide

Action: Fixed combination of TMP and SMZ, synthetic folate antagonists and enzyme inhibitors that prevent bacterial synthesis of essential nucleic acids and proteins; effective against *Pneumocystis carinii* pneumonitis, *Shigellosis enteritis,* most strains of *Enterobacteriaceae, Nocardia, Legionella micdadei,* and *Legionella pneumophila,* and *Haemophilus ducreyi*

Dose: 160 mg TMP/800 mg SMZ (DS) PO bid

Indication: For cellulitis, pneumonitis, enteritis, severe complicated UTIs, acute otitis media, acute episodes of chronic bronchitis, prevention of traveler's diarrhea, cholera

Contraindications: TMP, SMZ, sulfonamide, or bisulfite hypersensitivity; group A beta-hemolytic streptococcal pharyngitis; megaloblastic anemia due to folate deficiency; use caution with severe allergy or bronchial asthma, G6PD deficiency, and sulfonamide derivative drug (acetazolamide, thiazides, tolbutamide) hypersensitivity; pregnancy category C

Adverse Effects: Rash, toxic epidermal necrolysis; nausea, vomiting, diarrhea, anorexia, hepatitis, pseudomembranous enterocolitis, stomatitis, glossitis, abdominal pain; kidney failure, oliguria, anuria, crystalluria; agranulocytosis, aplastic anemia, megaloblastic anemia, hypoprothrombinemia, thrombocytopenia; weakness, arthralgia, myalgia, photosensitivity, allergic myocarditis

Interactions: May effect and toxicity of oral anticoagulants and methotrexate

28. ZOLPIDEM (AMBIEN) - CONTROLLED SUBSTANCE: SCHEDULE IV

Class: CNS agent – non-benzodiazepine; anxiolytic, sedative-hypnotic

Action: Nonbenzodiazepine hypnotic that does not have muscle relaxant or anticonvulsant effects; preserves deep sleep (stages 3 and 4) at hypnotic doses

Dose: 5–10 mg PO qhs, limited to 7–10 days

Indications: For short-term treatment of insomnia

Contraindications: Pregnancy category B

Adverse Effects: Headache on awakening, drowsiness or fatigue, lethargy, drugged feeling, depression, anxiety, irritability, dizziness, double vision; doses >10 mg may be associated with anterograde amnesia or memory impairment; dyspepsia, nausea, vomiting; myalgia

Interactions: CNS depressants, alcohol, and phenothiazines augment CNS depression; food significantly decreases extent and rate of absorption, do NOT give with or immediately after a meal

SECTION THREE

RMED PHARMACOLOGY
SECTION III

"FAMILIAR"

PHARMACOLOGY SECTION III: "FAMILIAR"

1.	AZITHROMYCIN (ZITHROMAX)	500 mg PO on day 1, then 250 mg qd x 4 days
2.	CELECOXIB (CELEBREX)	100–200 mg PO qd-bid
3.	CHLORPHENIRAMINE	2–4 mg PO tid-qid or 8–12 mg PO bid-tid
4.	CIPROFLOXACIN (CIPRO)	250-750 mg PO bid or 200-400 mg IV q8-12h
5.	CYCLOBENZAPRINE (FLEXERIL)	5–10 mg PO tid
6.	DICLOFENAC (VOLTAREN)	25-75mg PO bid-tid
7.	DOCUSATE (COLACE)	50–500 mg/day PO divided qd-qid
8.	HYDROCODONE (VICODIN w/ TYLENOL)	5–10 mg PO q4–6h
9.	KETOCONAZOLE (NIZORAL)	Topically, AAA qd-bid; 200–400 mg PO daily
10.	METHOCARBAMOL (ROBAXIN)	1.5 g PO qid x 2-3 d
11.	METHYLPREDNISOLONE (SOLU-MEDROL)	2–60 mg/d PO; 4–80 mg/wk IM; 10–250 mg IV
12.	METRONIDAZOLE (FLAGYL, METROGEL)	250 mg PO tid x 5-7 d; topically AAA bid
13.	MUPIROCIN (BACTROBAN)	topically AAA tid-qid
14.	NAPHAZOLINE (CLEAR EYES)	1 drop in each eye qid
15.	NAPROXEN (NAPROSYN)	250–500 mg PO bid (max: 1000 mg/d)
16.	OMEPRAZOLE (PRILOSEC)	20 mg PO qd
17.	OXYCODONE	5–10 mg PO q6h
18.	RABEPRAZOLE (ACIPHEX)	20 mg PO qd
19.	SCOPOLAMINE (TRANSDERM-SCOP)	transdermal patch behind ear 12 h before travel
20.	TERBINAFINE (LAMISIL)	topically AAA qd-bid; 250 mg PO qd
21.	TINIDAZOLE (TINDAMAX)	2 g PO qd
22.	TRAMADOL (ULTRAM)	50–100mg PO q4–6h prn (max: 400 mg/d)

1. AZITHROMYCIN (ZITHROMAX)

Class: Antimicrobial – antibiotic; macrolide

Action: Reversibly binds to 50S ribosomal subunit of susceptible organisms inhibiting protein synthesis; effective against mild to moderate infections caused by pyogenic streptococci, *Streptococcus pneumoniae, Haemophilus influenzae, Mycobacterium avium–intracellulare,* and *Staphylococcus aureus*

Dose: For most bacterial infections, 500 mg PO on day 1, then 250 mg qd x 4 days; for acute bacterial sinusitis, 500 mg qd x 3 days; for gonorrhea, 2 g PO as single dose

Indications: For pneumonia, lower respiratory tract infections, pharyngitis, tonsillitis, gonorrhea, nongonococcal urethritis, skin infections, otitis media, and acute bacterial sinusitis

Contraindications: Macrolide hypersensitivity; pregnancy category B

Adverse Effects: Headache, dizziness; nausea, vomiting, diarrhea, abdominal pain; hepatotoxicity

Interactions: Antacids may decrease peak level; may increase toxicity of ergotamine; food will decrease the amount of azithromycin absorbed by 50%

2. CELECOXIB (CELEBREX)

Class: CNS agent – COX-2 inhibitor; NSAID, anti-inflammatory, analgesic, antipyretic

Action: Inhibits prostaglandin synthesis by inhibiting cyclooxygenase-2 (COX-2); does not inhibit cyclooxygenase-1 (COX-1); reduces pain of rheumatoid and osteoarthritis

Dose: 100–200 mg PO qd-bid

Indications: For mild to moderate pain management, also used for osteoarthritis and rheumatoid arthritis

Contraindications: Celecoxib hypersensitivity; severe hepatic impairment; asthmatic patients with aspirin triad; advanced renal disease; concurrent use of diuretics and ACE inhibitors; anemia; pregnancy category C (D in 3rd trimester)

Adverse Effects: Back pain, peripheral edema; abdominal pain, diarrhea, dyspepsia, flatulence, nausea; dizziness, headache, insomnia; pharyngitis, rhinitis, sinusitis, rash

Interactions: May decrease effectiveness of ACE inhibitors; fluconazole and lithium increases concentrations; may increase INR with warfarin

3. CHLORPHENIRAMINE (+ SUDAFED = DECONAMINE)

Class: ENT agent – H_1-receptor antagonist, antihistamine

Dose: 2–4 mg PO tid-qid or 8–12 mg PO bid-tid (max: 24 mg/d)

Actions: Competes with histamine for H_1-receptor sites on effector cells; promotes capillary permeability, edema formation, and constrictive action on respiratory, gastrointestinal, and vascular smooth muscles

Indications: For symptomatic relief of uncomplicated allergic conditions, to prevent transfusion and drug reactions in susceptible patients, and as an adjunct to epinephrine and other standard measures in anaphylactic reactions

Contraindications: Antihistamine hypersensitivity, lower respiratory tract symptoms, narrow-angle glaucoma, obstructive prostatic hypertrophy or other bladder neck obstruction, GI obstruction or stenosis, MAOIs; pregnancy category B (D in 3rd trimester)

Adverse Effects: Sensation of chest tightness, palpitations, tachycardia, mild hypo- or hypertension; epigastric distress, anorexia, nausea, vomiting, constipation, diarrhea; drowsiness, sedation, headache, dizziness, vertigo, fatigue, disturbed coordination, tremors, euphoria, nervousness, restlessness, insomnia; dryness of mouth, nose, and throat; tinnitus, vertigo, acute labyrinthitis, thickened bronchial secretions, blurred vision, diplopia; urinary frequency or retention, dysuria.

Interactions: Alcohol and other CNS depressants produce additive sedation and CNS depression

4. CIPROFLOXACIN (CIPRO)

Class: Antimicrobial – antibiotic; quinolone

Action: Synthetic broad spectrum bactericidal agent; inhibits DNA-gyrase, an enzyme necessary for bacterial DNA replication, transcription, repair, recombination, and transposition; effective against many gram-positive and gram-negative organisms including *Citrobacter diversus, Enterobacter cloacae, Enterobacter aerogenes, Escherichia coli, Haemophilus influenzae, Klebsiella pneumoniae, Neisseria gonorrhoeae, Proteus mirabilis, Proteus vulgaris, Pseudomonas aeruginosa, Serratia marcescens, Staphylococcus aureus, Streptococcus pyogenes, Shigella,* and *Salmonella*; less active against gram-positive than gram-negative bacteria, although active against many gram-positive aerobic bacteria, including penicillinase-producing, non-penicillinase-producing, and methicillin-resistant *Staphylococci;* however, many strains of *Streptococci* are relatively resistant; inactive against most anaerobic bacteria; resistant to some strains of methicillin-resistant *Staphylococcus aureus* (MRSA)

Dose: 250-750 mg PO bid or 200-400 mg IV q8-12h

Indications: For infections of the lower respiratory tract, skin and skin structures, bone and joints, GI tract, urinary tract, prostate; also used for nosocomial pneumonia, acute sinusitis, and post-exposure prophylaxis for anthrax

Contraindications: Quinolone hypersensitivity; syphilis, viral infection; tendon inflammation or tendon pain; pregnancy category C

Adverse Effects: Nausea, vomiting, diarrhea, cramps, gas, pseudomembranous colitis; tendon rupture; headache, vertigo, malaise, peripheral neuropathy, seizures

Interactions: May increase theophylline levels; antacids, sulcralfate, iron decrease absorption; may increase PT for patients on warfarin; may cause false positive on opiate screening tests

5. CYCLOBENZAPRINE (FLEXERIL)

Class: Autonomic nervous system agent – central acting; skeletal muscle relaxant

Action: Structurally and pharmacologically related to TCAs; relieves skeletal muscle spasm of local origin without interfering with muscle function; believed to act primarily within CNS at brain stem with some action at spinal cord level; depresses tonic somatic motor activity, although both gamma and alpha motor neurons are affected; increases circulating norepinephrine by blocking synaptic reuptake, thus producing antidepressant effect; has sedative effect and potent central and peripheral anticholinergic activity

Dose: 5–10 mg PO tid prn muscle spasm (max: 60 mg/d); do not use longer than 2-3 wks

Indications: As adjunct to rest and physical therapy for short-term relief of muscle spasm associated with acute musculoskeletal conditions

Contraindications: Recovery phase of MI; cardiac arrhythmias, heart block or conduction disturbances; CHF, hyperthyroidism; pregnancy category B

Adverse Effects: Tongue and face edema, sweating, myalgia, hepatitis, alopecia; toxic potential of TCAs; tachycardia, syncope, palpitation, vasodilation, chest pain, orthostatic hypotension, dyspnea; arrhythmias; dry mouth, indigestion, unpleasant taste, coated or discolored tongue, vomiting, anorexia, abdominal pain, flatulence, diarrhea, paralytic ileus; drowsiness, dizziness, weakness, fatigue, asthenia, paresthesias, tremors, muscle twitching, insomnia, euphoria, disorientation, mania, ataxia; pruritus, urticaria, rash; increased or decreased libido, impotence

Interactions: Alcohol, barbiturates, other CNS depressants enhance CNS depression; potentiates anticholinergic effect of phenothiazine and other anticholinergics; MAOIs may precipitate hypertensive crisis

6. DICLOFENAC (VOLTAREN)

Class: CNS Agent – NSAID, anti-inflammatory, analgesic, antipyretic,

Action: Potent inhibitor of cyclooxygenase, decreases prostaglandin synthesis

Dose: 25-75mg PO bid-tid

Indications: For mild to moderate pain management, reduction of fever, and for symptomatic relief of rheumatoid arthritis, osteoarthritis, acute gout, bursitis, myalgias, sciatica, tendonitis, acute soft tissue injuries including sprains and strains, headache, migraines, dental and other minor surgical pain, photophobia associated with refractive surgery

Contraindications: NSAID or aspirin hypersensitivity, NSAID or aspirin induced asthma, urticaria, angioedema, bronchospasm, severe rhinitis, or shock; pregnancy category B

Adverse Effects: Dizziness, headache, drowsiness; tinnitus; rash, pruritus; dyspepsia, nausea, vomiting, abdominal pain, cramps, constipation, diarrhea, indigestion, abdominal distension, flatulence, peptic ulcer; increased LFTs; fluid retention, hypertension, CHF; asthma; back, leg, or joint pain; hyperglycemia; prolonged bleeding time, inhibits platelet aggregation

Interactions: Increases cyclosporine-induced nephrotoxicity; increases methotrexate, lithium, and digoxin levels and toxicity; may decrease BP-lowering effects of diuretics; herbals (feverfew, garlic, ginger, ginkgo) may increase risk of bleeding

7. DOCUSATE (COLACE)

Class: GI agent – stool softener

Action: Anionic surface-active agent with emulsifying and wetting properties; detergent action lowers surface tension, permitting water and fats to penetrate and soften stools for easier passage

Dose: 50–500 mg/day PO divided qd-qid

Indications: For treatment of constipation associated with hard and dry stools, also used prophylactically in patients taking narcotics or patients who should avoid straining during defecation

Contraindications: Atonic constipation, nausea, vomiting, abdominal pain, fecal impaction, structural anomalies of colon and rectum, intestinal obstruction or perforation; patients on sodium restriction or with renal dysfunction; concomitant use of mineral oil; pregnancy category C

Adverse Effects: Mild abdominal cramps, diarrhea, nausea, bitter taste; rash

Interactions: Increases systemic absorption of mineral oil

8. HYDROCODONE (VICODIN w/ TYLENOL) - CONTROLLED SUBSTANCE: SCHEDULE III

Class: CNS agent – narcotic (opiate) agonist; analgesic; antitussive

Action: Morphine derivative similar to codeine but more addicting and with slightly greater antitussive and analgesic effect; CNS depressant with moderate to severe relief of pain; suppresses cough reflex by direct action on cough center in medulla

Dose: 5–10 mg PO q4–6h prn (max: 15 mg/dose); common ingredient in a variety of proprietary mixtures, only available in the US as combination with other drugs

Indications: For moderate to severe pain management, and for hyperactive or nonproductive cough

Contraindications: Opiate hypersensitivity; pregnancy category C

Adverse Effects: Dry mouth, constipation, nausea, vomiting; light-headedness, sedation, dizziness, drowsiness, euphoria, dysphoria; respiratory depression; urticaria, rash, pruritus

Interactions: Alcohol, CNS depressants, and herbal (St. John's wort) increases CNS depression

9. KETOCONAZOLE (NIZORAL)

Class: Antimicrobial – antibiotic; imidazole antifungal

Action: Broad-spectrum antifungal that interferes with synthesis of ergosterol and results in an increase in cell membrane permeability; fungistatic, but may be fungicidal in high concentrations

Dose: Topically, AAA qd-bid; 200–400 mg PO qd (monitor baseline LFTs, repeat at least monthly)

Indications: Oral form for systemic fungal infections including candidiasis, oral thrush, histoplasmosis, coccidioidomycosis, paracoccidioidomycosis, blastomycosis, and chromomycosis; topical form for tinea corporis and tinea cruris (*Epidermophyton floccosum, Trichophyton mentagrophytes, Trichophyton rubrum*) and and tinea versicolor (*Malassezia furfur)*, seborrheic dermatitis

Contraindications: Ketoconazole hypersensitivity; alcoholism, fungal meningitis; onychomycosis; ocular administration; pregnancy category C

Adverse Effects: Rash, erythema, urticaria, pruritus, angioedema, anaphylaxis; nausea, vomiting, anorexia, epigastric or abdominal pain, constipation, diarrhea, fatal hepatic necrosis; gynecomastia; loss of libido, impotence, oligospermia, hair loss; acute hypoadrenalism, renal hypofunction

Interactions: Alcohol may cause sunburnlike reaction; antacids, anticholinergics, H2-receptor antagonists decrease absorption; isoniazid, rifampin increase metabolism and activity; levels of phenytoin and ketoconazole decreased; may increase cyclosporine and trazodone levels and toxicity; warfarin may potentiate hypoprothrombinemia; may increase levels of carbamazepine, cisapride, resulting in arrhythmias; may increase ergotamine toxicity; herbal echinacea may increase risk of hepatotoxicity

10. METHOCARBAMOL (ROBAXIN)

Class: Somatic nervous system agent – central-acting, skeletal muscle relaxant

Action: Exerts skeletal muscle relaxant action by depressing multisynaptic pathways in the spinal cord that control muscular spasm, and possibly by sedative effect; no direct action on skeletal muscles

Dose: 1.5 g PO qid x 2-3 d

Indications: For management of discomfort associated with acute musculoskeletal disorders as adjunct to physical therapy and other measures

Contraindications: Comatose; CNS depression; acidosis, kidney dysfunction; pregnancy category C

Adverse Effects: Fever, anaphylactic reaction, flushing, syncope, convulsions; urticaria, pruritus, rash, thrombophlebitis, pain, sloughing; conjunctivitis, blurred vision, nasal congestion; drowsiness, dizziness, light-headedness, headache; hypotension, bradycardia; nausea, metallic taste

Interactions: Alcohol and other CNS depressants enhance CNS depression

11. METHYLPREDNISOLONE (SOLU-MEDROL)

Class: Hormones and synthetic substitutes – adrenal corticosteroid, glucosteroid, antiinflammatory

Action: Intermediate-acting synthetic steroid with less sodium and water retention effects than hydrocortisone; inhibits phagocytosis and release of allergic substances; modifies immune response to various stimuli; antiinflammatory and immunosuppressive

Dose: For inflammation, 2–60 mg/d PO; 4–80 mg/wk IM (Acetate) for 1–4 wk; 10–250 mg IV (Succinate) q6h; for acute spinal cord injury, 30 mg/kg IV over 15 min, followed in 45 min by 5.4 mg/kg/h x 23h

Indications: For management of acute and chronic inflammatory diseases, control of severe acute and chronic allergic processes, acute bronchial asthma, prevention of fat embolism in patient with long-bone fracture

Contraindications: Systemic fungal infections; pregnancy category C

Adverse Effects: Euphoria, headache, insomnia, confusion, psychosis; CHF, edema, nausea, vomiting, peptic ulcer; muscle weakness, delayed wound healing, muscle wasting, osteoporosis, aseptic necrosis of bone, spontaneous fractures; cushingoid features, growth suppression in children, carbohydrate intolerance, hyperglycemia; cataracts; leukocytosis; hypokalemia

Interactions: Amphotericin B, furosemide, thiazide diuretics increase potassium loss; may enhance virus replication or increase attenuated virus vaccine adverse effects; isoniazid, phenytoin, phenobarbital, rifampin increase metabolism and decrease effectiveness

12. METRONIDAZOLE (FLAGYL, METROGEL)

Class: Antimicrobial – antibiotic, antitrichomonal, amebicide

Action: Synthetic compound with direct trichomonacidal, amebicidal, and antibacterial activity (anaerobic bacteria and some gram-negative bacteria); effective against *Trichomonas vaginalis, Entamoeba histolytica, Giardia lamblia*, obligate anaerobic bacteria, gram-negative anaerobic bacilli, and *Clostridia*; microaerophilic *Streptococci* and most aerobic bacteria are resistant

Dose: For giardia 250 mg PO tid x 5-7 d; for amebiasis 500–750 mg PO tid; for pseudomembranous colitis, 250–500 mg PO tid-qid; for trichomoniasis, 2 g PO once; for rosacea, topically AAA bid

Indications: For giardiasis, trichomoniasis, amebiasis, and amebic liver abscess; topical for rosacea

Contraindications: Blood dyscrasias; active CNS disease; pregnancy category B

Adverse Effects: hypersensitivity (rash, urticaria, pruritus, flushing), fever, fleeting joint pains, *Candida* overgrowth; vertigo, headache, ataxia, confusion, irritability, depression, restlessness, weakness, fatigue, drowsiness, insomnia, paresthesias, sensory neuropathy; nausea, vomiting, anorexia, epigastric distress, abdominal cramps, diarrhea, constipation, dry mouth, metallic or bitter taste, proctitis; polyuria, dysuria, pyuria, incontinence, cystitis, decreased libido, nasal congestion; ECG changes (flattening of T wave)

Interactions: Oral anticoagulants potentiate hypoprothrombinemia; alcohol and solutions of citalopram, ritonavir, lopinavir, and IV formulations of sulfamethoxazole, trimethoprim, nitroglycerin may elicit disulfiram reaction due to the alcohol content; disulfiram causes acute psychosis; phenobarbital increases metabolism; may increase lithium levels; fluorouracil, azathioprine may cause transient neutropenia

13. MUPIROCIN (BACTROBAN)

Class: Antimicrobial – antibiotic; pseudomonic acid

Action: Topical antibacterial produced by fermentation of *Pseudomonas fluorescens*; inhibits protein synthesis by binding with bacterial transfer-RNA; effective against *Staphylococcus aureus* [including methicillin-resistant (MRSA) and beta-lactamase-producing strains], *Staphylococcus epidermidis, Staphylococcus saprophyticus,* and *Streptococcus pyogenes*

Dose: Topically AAA tid-qid x 1-2 wks

Indications: For impetigo or nasal carriage due to *Staphylococcus aureus*, beta-hemolytic Streptococci, and *Streptococcus pyogenes*; superficial skin infections

Contraindications: Hypersensitivity to any of its components; pregnancy category B

Adverse Effects: Burning, stinging, pain, pruritus, rash, erythema, dry skin, tenderness, swelling; intranasal, local stinging, soreness, dry skin, pruritus

Interactions: Incompatible with salicylic acid 2%; do not mix in hydrophilic vehicles or coal tar solutions; chloramphenicol may interfere with bactericidal action

14. NAPHAZOLINE (NAPHCON, VASOCON, CLEAR EYES)

Class: Autonomic nervous system agent – sympathomimetic, alpha-adrenergic agonist, vasoconstrictor, decongestant

Action: Direct-acting imidazoline derivative with marked alpha-adrenergic activity; systemic absorption may cause CNS depression rather than stimulation; produces rapid and prolonged vasoconstriction of arterioles, decreasing fluid exudation and mucosal engorgement

Dose: 1 drop in each eye qid prn for up to 4 days

Indications: For ocular vasoconstriction and decongestion

Contraindications: Narrow-angle glaucoma; MAOIs, TCAs; pregnancy category C

Adverse Effects: Hypersensitivity reactions, headache, nausea, weakness, sweating, drowsiness, hypothermia, coma; hypertension, bradycardia, shock-like hypotension; increased IOP, rebound congestion and chemical rhinitis with frequent and continued use

Interactions: TCAs and maprotiline may potentiate pressor effects

15. NAPROXEN (NAPROSYN)

Class: CNS agent – NSAID; anti-inflammatory, analgesic, antipyretic

Action: Propionic acid derivative with properties similar to ibuprofen; inhibits prostaglandin synthesis and platelet aggregation; prolongs bleeding time

Dose: 250–500 mg PO bid (max: 1000 mg/d)

Indications: For mild to moderate pain management and symptomatic treatment of acute and chronic arthritis

Contraindications: peptic ulcer; history of asthma, rhinitis, urticaria, bronchospasm, or shock precipitated by aspirin or other NSAIDs; pregnancy category B

Adverse Effects: Headache, drowsiness, dizziness, lightheadedness, depression; palpitation, dyspnea, peripheral edema, CHF, tachycardia; blurred vision, tinnitus, hearing loss; anorexia, heartburn, indigestion, nausea, vomiting, thirst, GI bleeding, elevated LFTs; thrombocytopenia, leukopenia, eosinophilia, pruritus, rash, ecchymosis; nephrotoxicity; pulmonary edema

Interactions: Herbals (feverfew, garlic, ginger, ginkgo) may increase bleeding

16. OMEPRAZOLE (PRILOSEC)

Class: GI agent – proton pump inhibitor (PPI)

Action: Antisecretory compound that is a gastric acid pump inhibitor; suppresses gastric acid secretion by inhibiting the H^+, K^+-ATPase enzyme system [the acid (proton H^+) pump] in the parietal cells which relieves gastrointestinal distress and promotes ulcer healing

Dose: 20 mg PO qd x 4–8 wk

Indications: For treatment of duodenal and gastric ulcers, gastroesophageal reflux disease, and erosive esophagitis; used in combination with clarithromycin and metronidazole to treat duodenal ulcers associated with *Helicobacter pylori*

Contraindications: PPI hypersensitivity, GI bleeding, pregnancy category C

Adverse Effects: Headache, dizziness, fatigue; diarrhea, abdominal pain, nausea; hematuria, proteinuria; rash

Interactions: May increase diazepam, phenytoin, and warfarin levels

17. OXYCODONE - CONTROLLED SUBSTANCE: SCHEDULE II

Class: CNS agent – narcotic (opiate) agonist; analgesic

Action: Opium alkaloid semisynthetic derivative with action and potency similar to morphine; binds with stereo-specific receptors in various sites of CNS altering both pain perception and emotional response

Dose: 5–10 mg PO q6h prn

Indications: For moderate to moderately severe pain management; more effective in acute than chronic pain; used for bursitis, dislocations, simple fractures, other injuries, neuralgia, and postoperative pain

Contraindications: Oxycodone hypersensitivity; pregnancy category B (D for prolonged use or high dose use at term)

Adverse Effects: Euphoria, dysphoria, light-headedness, dizziness, sedation, anorexia, nausea, vomiting, constipation, jaundice; shortness of breath, respiratory depression; pruritus, rash; bradycardia; unusual bleeding or bruising; dysuria, urinary frequency and retention

Interactions: Alcohol, CNS depressants, and herbal (St. John's wort) add to CNS depressant activity

18. RABEPRAZOLE (ACIPHEX)

Class: GI agent – proton pump inhibitor (PPI)

Action: Gastric PPI that specifically suppresses gastric acid secretion by inhibiting the H^+, K^+-ATPase enzyme system (the acid [proton H^+] pump) in the parietal cells of the stomach; does not exhibit H_2-histamine receptor antagonist properties

Dose: 20 mg PO qd

Indications: For healing and maintenance of erosive or ulcerative gastroesophageal reflux disease (GERD), duodenal ulcers, and hypersecretory conditions

Contraindications: PPI hypersensitivity; pregnancy category B

Adverse Effects: Headache; Stevens-Johnson syndrome, toxic epidermal necrolysis, erythema multiforme

Interactions: May decrease absorption of ketoconazole; may increase digoxin levels

19. SCOPOLAMINE (TRANSDERM-SCOP)

Class: Autonomic nervous system agent – parasympatholytic; anticholinergic, antimuscarinic, antispasmodic

Action: Alkaloid of belladonna with peripheral action resembling those of atropine, but in contrast, produces CNS depression with marked sedative and tranquilizing effects for use in anesthesia; potent mydriatic and cycloplegic action inhibiting secretions of salivary, bronchial, and sweat glands with less prominent effect on heart, intestines, and bronchial muscles

Dose: For motion sickness, 0.25–0.6 mg PO 1 h before travel or topical transdermal disc patch applied to dry surface behind ear q72h starting 12 h before travel; for ophthalmic refraction 1–2 drops in eye 1 h prior; for pre-anesthesia PO 0.5-1 mg PO or 0.3-0.6 mg IM/SC/IV

Indications: Prophylactic agent for motion sickness; used as mydriatic and cycloplegic in ophthalmology; preanesthetic agent to control bronchial, nasal, pharyngeal and salivary secretions; control of spasticity and drooling in paralytic and spastic states

Contraindications: Anticholinergic, belladonna, or barbiturate hypersensitivity; asthma; hepatitis; narrow angle glaucoma; GI or GU obstructive diseases; myasthenia gravis; pregnancy category C

Adverse Effects: Fatigue, dizziness, drowsiness, disorientation, restlessness, hallucinations, toxic psychosis; dry mouth and throat, constipation; urinary retention; decreased heart rate; dilated pupils, photophobia, blurred vision, follicular conjunctivitis; depressed respiration; local irritation, rash

Interactions: Amantadine, antihistamines, TCAs, quinidine, disopyramide, procainamide add to anticholinergic effects; decreases levodopa effects; methotrimeprazine may precipitate extrapyramidal effects; decreases absorption and antipsychotic effects of phenothiazines

20. TERBINAFINE (LAMISIL)

Class: Antimicrobial – antibiotic; antifungal

Action: Inhibits sterol biosynthesis in fungi; ergosterol, the principal sterol in the fungal cell membrane, becomes depleted and interferes with cell membrane function, thus producing antifungicidal effect

Dose: For tinea pedis, tinea cruris, and tinea corporis, topically AAA qd-bid x 1-7 wks; for onychomycosis, 250 mg PO qd x 6 wks for fingernails 12 wks for toenails (monitor baseline LFTs, repeat at least monthly)

Indications: For topical treatment of superficial mycoses such as interdigital tinea pedis, tinea cruris, and tinea corporis due to *Epidermophyton floccosum, Trichophyton mentagrophytes*, or *T. rubrum*; for oral treatment of onychomycosis due to tinea unguium

Contraindications: Terbinafine hypersensitivity; pregnancy category B

Adverse Effects: Pruritus, local burning, dryness, rash, vesiculation, redness, contact dermatitis at application site; headache; diarrhea, dyspepsia, abdominal pain, neutropenia; taste disturbances

Interactions: May increase theophylline levels; may decrease cyclosporine and rifampin levels

21. TINIDAZOLE (TINDAMAX)

Class: Antimicrobial – azole antibiotic; antiprotozoal amebicide

Action: Made from cell extracts of *Trichomonas*, the free radicals generated may be responsible for antiprotozoal activity; effective against *Trichomonas vaginalis*, *Giardia duodenalis*, *Entamoeba histolytica*

Dose: Giardiasis 2 g PO x 1 dose or Amebiasis/Amebic liver abscess 2 g PO qd x 3-5d, take with food

Indications: For treatment of protozoa infections (giardiasis, amebiasis, amebic liver abscess, trichomoniasis)

Contraindications: azole antibiotic hypersensitivity; pregnancy category D (1st trimester) and C (2nd/3rd)

Adverse Effects: Weakness, fatigue, malaise; dizziness, headache; metallic/bitter taste, nausea, anorexia, dyspepsia, cramps, epigastric discomfort, vomiting, constipation

Interactions: May increase INR with warfarin; alcohol may cause abdominal cramps, nausea, vomiting, headache, flushing; psychotic reactions with disulfiram; may increase half-life of phenytoin; may increase level and toxicity of lithium, fluorouracil, cyclosporine, tacrolimus; cholestyramine may reduce absorption

22. TRAMADOL (ULTRAM)

Class: CNS agent – narcotic (opiate) agonist; analgesic

Action: Centrally acting opiate receptor agonist that inhibits uptake of norepinephrine and serotonin, suggesting both opioid and nonopioid mechanisms of pain relief; may produce opioid-like effects, but causes less respiratory depression than morphine

Dose: 50–100mg PO q4–6h prn (max: 400 mg/d); may start with 25 mg/d if not well tolerated, and increase by 25 mg q3d up to 200 mg/d

Indications: For management of moderate to moderately severe pain

Contraindications: Opioid analgesic or tramadol hypersensitivity; MAOIs; acute alcohol intoxication, hypnotics, centrally acting analgesics, opioids, psychotropics; substance abuse; pregnancy category C

Adverse Effects: Drowsiness, dizziness, vertigo, fatigue, headache, somnolence, restlessness, euphoria, confusion, anxiety, coordination disturbance, sleep disturbance, seizures; palpitations, vasodilation; nausea, vomiting, diarrhea, constipation, xerostoma, dyspepsia, abdominal pain, anorexia, flatulence; sweating, anaphylaxis, withdrawal syndrome with abrupt discontinuation; rash; visual disturbances; urinary retention/frequency

Interactions: Carbamazepine significantly decreases levels; may increase adverse effects of MAOIs, TCAs, cyclobenzaprine, phenothiazines, SSRIs; MAOIs may enhance seizure risk; may increase CNS effects when used with other CNS depressants; herbal St. John's wort may increase sedation

SECTION FOUR

RMED MEDICAL OPERATIONS & PLANNING

SENIOR MEDIC DUTIES AND RESPONSIBILITIES

The senior medic is customarily known as a company senior medic, and he traditionally functions in the capacity of a squad leader. However, in the context of the Ranger Medic Handbook the senior medic duty description will be used to define the responsibilities of the highest ranking and most experienced medic present at any given location and time. This medic is designated as the "senior medic" at that specific location and thus is responsible for the duties and responsibilities as listed below.

❖ **Principal medical advisor to the commander and senior enlisted advisor**

❖ **Provide and supervise advanced trauma management within protocols and sick call within scope-of-practice**

❖ **Lead, supervise, and train junior medics**
  ➢ Individual training
  ➢ Health and welfare
  ➢ Development and counseling
  ➢ Troop leading procedures and pre-combat inspections (PCIs)

❖ **Plan, supervise, and conduct casualty response training for Rangers and Leaders**
  ➢ Ranger First Responder (RFR)
  ➢ Casualty Response Training for Ranger Leaders (CRTRL)
  ➢ Opportunity Training / Spot-Checking

❖ **Maintain company level medical equipment and supplies**
  ➢ Accountability / Inventory
  ➢ Maintenance / Serviceability
  ➢ PCI of Individual Ranger Bleeding Control Kits
  ➢ PCI of Squad Casualty Response Kits
  ➢ Requisition and Receive Class VIII (Medical Supplies) from appropriate source

❖ **Plan, coordinate, and execute medical planning for company level operations**
  ➢ On-Target casualty response plan
  ➢ CASEVAC from target to next higher medical capability
  ➢ Task organization of company medics

❖ **Conduct after action reviews and report and archive medical lessons learned**

❖ **Monitor the status of health in the unit / element**
  ➢ Physically Limiting Profiles
  ➢ Command Health Report
  ➢ MEDPROS Data Entry and Information Review

MEDICAL & CASUALTY RESPONSE PLANNING
PART 1: Initial Planning / WARNORD

1-A. MEDICAL THREAT ASSESSMENT
- ☐ AFMIC CD – Find Country / Area of Operations
  - ✦ Host Country (ISB / FSB)
  - ✦ Target Country
- ☐ Determine known health threats & risks
  - ✦ Diseases / Illnesses
  - ✦ Environmental threats (Plants, Animals, Climate, Terrain)
- ☐ Current Unit SRP Status
- ☐ Preventive Medicine Guidelines (what is required before, during, and after)
- ☐ Enemy weapons, munitions, and tactics, to include NBC?
- ☐ How ready is the unit if it encounters diseases / illnesses?
- ☐ What preparation is needed by the unit?
- ☐ Do Rangers need special preventive medicine items issued?

1-B. HIGHER MEDICAL GUIDELINES & REQUIREMENTS
- ☐ Chemoprophylaxis
  - ✦ Anti-Malarial Drugs
  - ✦ Other preventive measures
- ☐ Special SRP requirements
- ☐ WHO Traveler Advisory
- ☐ USSOCOM / USASOC / Theater guidelines
- ☐ Regiment / Battalion guidelines
- ☐ Do we need to change anything in the way we normally do business?

1-C. REQUESTS FOR INFORMATION (RFI)
- ☐ Request updates to AFMIC information
- ☐ Maps / Imagery
- ☐ Host Nation (ISB) Medical Capabilities
  - ✦ Hospitals / medical facilities
  - ✦ Nationwide medical training / competency
- ☐ Any information not covered in AFMIC-CD or higher guidelines
- ☐ Submit through medical, intelligence (S2), and/or operations (S3) channels
- ☐ Ask for more information for what you need to know

1-D. DETERMINE MEDICAL ASSETS
- ☐ Organic, Attached, Air, Ground, Theater, JTF, Host Nation, ISB, FSB, etc...
- ☐ CASEVAC / MEDEVAC Support
  - ✦ How many and what type?
  - ✦ Capabilities and Limitations?
  - ✦ Hoist and high angle extraction?
  - ✦ Medical Personnel and Equipment on board? Level of Training?

□ Determine nearest surgical capability
  + Where are your casualties being evacuated to?
  + What are the capabilities / limitations?
  + What is their MASCAL or overload for their system?
□ Determine Staging Base area medical support
  + Can they provide labs, x-rays, medications, preventive medicine, etc?

1-E. FAMILIARIZATION WITH MEDICAL ASSETS
□ Published References (Look it up!)
  + What is a CSH?
  + What is a FST?
  + What is an ASMC?
□ Can you see their layout / equipment?
□ Can you conduct familiarization training as required?
□ What are their capabilities and limitations?
□ Can you talk to them and what can <u>they</u> know about you and your mission?

PART 2: Tactical Operation Development

2-A. CASUALTY ESTIMATION
□ Look at the target and the templated enemy positions
□ Look at the commander's assault plan
□ Utilize Medical Course of Action Tool (MCOAT)
□ **Plan to take casualties during every phase of the operation (infiltration, assault, clear/secure, consolidate, defend, exfiltration).**
  + Where do you foresee taking casualties?
  + Where is it most critical for the medics to be located?
  + Do you need to task organize your medical team?
  + Where does the unit need to establish CCP's?
  + What evacuation methods need to be considered?
  + Where is the closest HLZ or AXP?
  + Where do you emplace and preposition medical assets/augmentation?
□ Review Preventive Medicine issues and anticipate DNBI
  + What are the health threats?
  + What actions will prevent or decrease disease and non-battle injuries?

2-B. DETERMINE KEY LOCATIONS
□ Based on your casualty estimation and the tactical assault plan...
  + Where should the CCP be located?
  + Where should patient exchanges be located? (CEP, CCP, HLZ, AXP)
  + Where are the projected blocking positions, fighting positions, etc...?
  + Where is the CP / TOC?
  + Who is in charge of each key location?
  + Primary and Alternate Locations?
  + What are the ground movement routes?

2-C. DETERMINE CASUALTY FLOW
- ☐ Point-of-Injury to Fixed Facility
- ☐ Where are your casualties being evacuated to?
  - ✦ Are you evacuating by ground or air to JCCP?
  - ✦ Are you evacuating by ground or air to an AXP/HLZ?
  - ✦ What are the distances and time of travel?
  - ✦ Can your patients make it that far? What needs to be corrected?
  - ✦ Who is evacuating your casualties?

EXAMPLE:

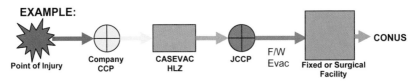

Point of Injury — Company CCP — CASEVAC HLZ — JCCP — F/W Evac — Fixed or Surgical Facility — CONUS

2-D. AIR CASEVAC PLAN
- ☐ What is the type of Air CASEVAC mission?
  - ✦ Dedicated – an air asset whose purpose after infiltration is casualty evacuation. It is outfitted and manned for casualty management
  - ✦ Designated – an air asset that will be the aircraft instructed to evacuate casualties. May be equipped for casualties if requested.
  - ✦ On-Call – air assets that are held in reserve or must be launched to respond to casualty evacuation. May also apply to MEDEVAC covering the area.
- ☐ Aircraft type?
- ☐ Maximum casualty load?
- ☐ How are casualties to be loaded?
  - ✦ Packaging requirements: Litters, Skedcos, etc..?
  - ✦ Is the aircraft equipped with litter stanchions?
  - ✦ Loading procedures? Approach procedures?
- ☐ What medical capability is on the aircraft?
  - ✦ Flight medic or medical officer?
  - ✦ Casualty management equipment?
  - ✦ Medical resupply bundles?
- ☐ Request Procedures?
  - ✦ Procedures for requesting CASEVAC?
  - ✦ 9-Line MEDEVAC request versus modified format?
  - ✦ Communication requirements?
- ☐ Launch Authority?
  - ✦ Who is the launch authority for the aircraft?
  - ✦ What are the impacts on Ranger CASEVAC operations?
- ☐ Landing requirements?
  - ✦ Special HLZ considerations?
  - ✦ Special markings required?
  - ✦ Special equipment required?

2-E. GROUND CASEVAC PLAN---TWO PHASES:
1. **Actions required on the target.**
2. **Actions required for evacuation away from the target.**
- ☐ How should Rangers move casualties on the target to the CCP?
  - ✦ Aid & Litter Teams
  - ✦ Skedco, Litter, etc...
  - ✦ Ranger Ground Mobility (Quad, GMV, RSOV)
- ☐ What is the type of Ground CASEVAC mission?
  - ✦ Dedicated – a ground asset whose purpose after infiltration is casualty evacuation. It is outfitted and manned for casualty management
  - ✦ Designated – a ground asset that will be the vehicles instructed to evacuate casualties. May be equipped for casualties if requested.
  - ✦ On-Call – ground assets that are held in reserve or must be launched to respond to casualty evacuation. This may be vehicles of opportunity (tactical or captured).
- ☐ Vehicle type and maximum casualty load?
- ☐ How are casualties to be loaded?
  - ✦ Packaging requirements: Litters, Skedcos, etc..?
  - ✦ Is the vehicle equipped with a carrying configuration?
  - ✦ Loading procedures?
- ☐ What medical capability is on the vehicle?
  - ✦ Medics? Medical Officers?
  - ✦ Casualty management equipment?
- ☐ Request Procedures?
  - ✦ Procedures for requesting ground CASEVAC?
  - ✦ 9-Line MEDEVAC request versus modified format?
  - ✦ Communication requirements?
- ☐ Launch Authority?
  - ✦ Who is the launch authority for the vehicles?
- ☐ Link-up Requirements
  - ✦ At your CCP or an AXP?
  - ✦ Marking / signaling procedures?

2-F. COMMUNICATIONS REQUIREMENTS
- ☐ Do all medics have radios?
- ☐ Can a medic contact a higher care provider for guidance?
- ☐ Types of radios / COMSEC?
- ☐ Medical Command & Control Delineation
- ☐ Callsigns / Frequencies / SOI
- ☐ Evacuation request frequencies?
- ☐ Evacuation asset frequencies?
- ☐ Casualty reporting/accountability?
- ☐ Re-Supply requests

2-G. CLASS VIII RE-SUPPLY REQUIREMENTS & METHODS
- ☐ How do you request re-supply?
- ☐ What are the re-supply methods?

+ Speedballs?
+ Drag-off bundles?
+ CDS?
☐ Medical packing lists? Do you need to reconfigure/repack (aidbag, pelican)?
☐ How do you request specific line items?

PART 3: Coordination & Synchronization

3-A. PLANNING INTERACTION (WHO TO TALK & COORDINATE WITH)
☐ Commander & Operations Officer (Tactical Plan)
☐ Executive Officer (Support & Resources)
☐ First Sergeant (CCP Operations, Manifests, Aid & Litter Teams)
☐ Battalion Medical Planner (Medical Aspects)
☐ Platoon Sergeants (Squad Casualty Response & CCPs)
☐ Junior Medics (Understanding of the Plan)
☐ Battalion Staff Planners
   + S1 Personnel (Casualty Tracking and Accountability)
   + S2 Intel (Health Threat/Intelligence Information)
   + S3 Air (Air CASEVAC Operations)
   + S4 Logistics (Ground CASEVAC & Re-Supply)
   + S6 Commo (Radios, Freqs, Callsigns)

PART 4: Briefs, Rehearsals, and Inspections

4-A. MEDICAL & CASUALTY RESPONSE OPORD BRIEFING AGENDA
☐ Health Threat
☐ Casualty Response Concept of the Operation
☐ Casualty Flow
☐ Key Locations (CCPs, HLZs, AXPs, etc)
☐ Requesting Procedures (CASEVAC, MEDEVAC, Assistance, Re-Supply)
☐ Medic callsigns / frequencies
☐ Casualty Accountability

4-B. BACK-BRIEF WITH JUNIOR MEDICS
☐ Ensure junior medics understand tactical plan AND casualty response plan
☐ Understand packaging requirements
☐ Understand casualty marking procedures
☐ Understand communications methods

4-C. REHEARSALS
☐ RFR Drills
☐ Squad Casualty Response Drills (care under fire, CASEVAC request/loading)
☐ Aid & Litter Team Drills
☐ CCP Operations (Assembly, security & movement, casualty movement, CCP

markings, vehicle parking, link-up procedures, casualty tracking & recording, triage, treatment and management of casualties)
- ☐ Evacuation Request and Loading Procedures
- ☐ COMMEX
- ☐ Casualty Tracking / Accountability

4-D. PRE-COMBAT INSPECTIONS
- ☐ Individual Rangers
  - ✦ Bleeding Control Kits (BCKs)
  - ✦ Preventive Medicine (Iodine Tabs, Doxycycline, Diamox, etc...)
- ☐ Squad Casualty Response Kit
  - ✦ Fire Team IV Kit
  - ✦ RFR Bags
  - ✦ Evacuation Equipment (Skedco, Litters, etc...)
  - ✦ Vehicle mounted aidbags
- ☐ RMED Aidbags (Pack and/or reconfigure as required)
  - ✦ Select appropriate aidbag system per mission requirements
  - ✦ Ensure packing list IAW recommended DOS stockage
- ☐ Re-Supply Packages (Pack and/or reconfigure per mission requirements)
  - ✦ Reconfigure per mission specifics (ground, air, etc...)
  - ✦ Utilize speedballs, bundles, or pull-off configured as required
  - ✦ Pre-position as required with aircraft and vehicles or at staging base with BLOC and logistics teams
- ☐ RMED Individual Equipment (weapon, NVG, radio, packing list, mission specific)
- ☐ Evacuation Assets (Quads, Vehicles, etc...)

PART 5: After Action Review in Training or Combat

- ☐ Was the mission executed as planned?
- ☐ What went right?
- ☐ What went wrong?
- ☐ What could have been done better?
- ☐ What could be fixed by planning / preparation?
- ☐ What could be fixed by training?
- ☐ What could be fixed by equipment modification?
- ☐ Identify and record Sustains & Improves by Phase of the Operation.

CASUALTY COLLECTION POINT (CCP) OPERATIONS

PART 1: Duties and Responsibilities

COMPANY MEDICS
❖ **Planning Phase**
  ➢ Provide recommendations and advise to leadership on medical support
  ➢ Medical Support Planning by phase of the operation
  ➢ Casualty Response & Evacuation Plan by phase of the operation
  ➢ Recommend to the Unit Leadership & Coordinate as required:
    • CCP Locations by phase
    • Medical Task Organization & Distribution
    • Ground (on the target) Evacuation Plan & Assets
    • Air/Ground (off the target) Evacuation Plan & Assets
    • CCP, HLZ, and Evacuation Asset Security
  ➢ Pre-Combat Inspections of Junior Medics, Squad Casualty Response Kits, and Individual Ranger BCK/RFR Tasks
❖ **Execution Phase**
  ➢ Triage, Treatment, Monitoring, and Packaging
  ➢ Delegation of Treatment
  ➢ Request Assistance from other medical or unit assets
  ➢ Provide guidance and recommendations to leadership on casualty management & evacuation

BATTALION MEDICAL PERSONNEL & MEDICAL PLANNERS
❖ **Planning Phase**
  ➢ Provide recommendations and advise to leadership on medical support
  ➢ Recommend to the Unit Leadership & Coordinate as required:
    • CCP Locations of subordinate units by phase
    • Medical Task Organization & Distribution
    • Ground (on the target) Evacuation Plan & Assets for all targets
    • Air/Ground (off the target) Evacuation Plan & Assets for all targets
    • CCP, HLZ, and Evacuation Asset Security for all targets
  ➢ Augmentation requirements of subordinate units
  ➢ Link-in with tactical operations
❖ **Execution Phase**
  ➢ Triage, Treatment, Monitoring, and Packaging
  ➢ Delegation of Treatment
  ➢ Request Assistance from other medical or platoon assets
  ➢ Provide guidance and recommendations to leadership on casualty management

UNIT LEADERSHIP

❖ **Planning Phase**
- ➤ Evacuation Plan by phase of the operation
- ➤ CCP locations, HLZ/AXP locations,
- ➤ Security of CCP, Security of HLZ/AXP
- ➤ Allocate Aid & Litter teams and carry evacuation equipment
- ➤ Accountability / Reporting Plan
- ➤ Distribution/Task Organization of Medical Personnel
- ➤ Pre-Combat Inspections of Junior Medics, Squad Casualty Response Kits, and Individual Ranger BCK/RFR Tasks
- ➤ Conduct Casualty Response Rehearsals

❖ **Execution Phase**
- ➤ Establish and Secure CCP
- ➤ Provide assistance to medics with EMT augmentation and directing aid & litter teams
- ➤ Gather and Distribute casualty equipment and sensitive items
- ➤ Accountability and Reporting to Higher
- ➤ Request Evacuation and Establish CASEVAC link-up point
- ➤ Manage KIA remains

PART 2: Casualty Response Rehearsals

- ➤ Critical in pre-mission planning and overall unit rehearsals
- ➤ Each element should rehearse alerting aid & litter team and movement of a casualty
  - Alert and movement
  - Evacuation equipment prep
  - Clearing / securing weapons
- ➤ CCP members rehearse the following:
  - Clear and Secure CCP Location
  - Choke Point / Triage
  - Marking & Tagging
  - Accountability & Reporting
  - Equipment removal tagging/consolidation

PART 3: CCP Site Selection

- ➤ Reasonably close to the fight
- ➤ Near templated areas of expected high casualties
- ➤ Cover and Concealment
- ➤ In building or on hardstand (exclusive CCP building limits confusion)
- ➤ Access to evacuation routes (foot, vehicle, aircraft)
- ➤ Proximity to Lines of Drift on the objective

- ➢ Adjacent to Objective Choke Points (breeches, HLZ's, etc...)
- ➢ Avoid natural or enemy choke points
- ➢ Area allowing passive security (inside the perimeter)
- ➢ Good Drainage
- ➢ Trafficable to evacuation assets
- ➢ Expandable if casualty load increases

PART 4: CCP Operational Guidelines

- ➢ 1SG / PSG is responsible for casualty flow and everything outside the CCP
  - Provides for CCP structure and organization (color coded with chemlights)
  - Maintains C2 and battlefield situational awareness
  - Controls aid & litter teams, and provides security
  - Strips, bags, tags, organizes, and maintains casualty equipment outside of treatment area as possible
  - Accountable for tracking casualties and equipment into and out of CCP and provides reports to higher
  - Casualties move through CCP entrance / exit choke point which should be marked with an IR Chemlight
- ➢ Medical personnel are responsible for everything inside the CCP
  - Triage officer sorts and organizes casualties at choke point into appropriate treatment categories
  - Medical officers and medics organize medical equipment and supplies and render treatment to casualties
  - EMTs, RFRs, A&L Teams assist with treatment and packaging of casualties
- ➢ Minimal casualties should remain with original element or assist with CCP security if possible
- ➢ KIAs should remain with original element or be transported to the BLOC

PART 5: CCP Building Guidelines

- ➢ Ensure building is cleared and secured
- ➢ Enter and assess the building prior to receiving casualties
  - Use largest rooms
  - Consider litter / skedco movement (can you do it in the area?)
  - Separate rooms for treatment categories?
  - Determine location of choke point / triage
  - Minimize congestion
- ➢ Remove / re-locate furniture or obstructions
- ➢ Color-code rooms to treatment categories (mark doors, etc...)

PART 6: Evacuation Guidelines

- ➢ Know the Evacuation Asset
  - Medical provider on board?
  - Monitoring equipment on board?
  - How many CAX can evacuate on asset?
- ➢ Packaging requirements for asset
  - Type litters?
  - Are there stirrups? Floor-Loading?
- ➢ Determine flow of casualties to the asset
  - Large Asset (Multiple CAX)
    - o Routine on first
    - o Priority on next
    - o Critical (Urgent) on last, so they are first off at destination
  - Small Asset
    - o Critical (Urgent) and Priority evacuated first

PART 7: CCP Layout Templates

- ➢ Use as a TEMPLATE
- ➢ Use as a Guideline
- ➢ Modify based on the objective and circumstances

CCP / CEP Template 1
(Adjacent to Breech)

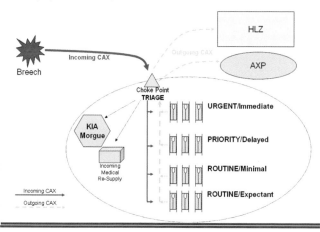

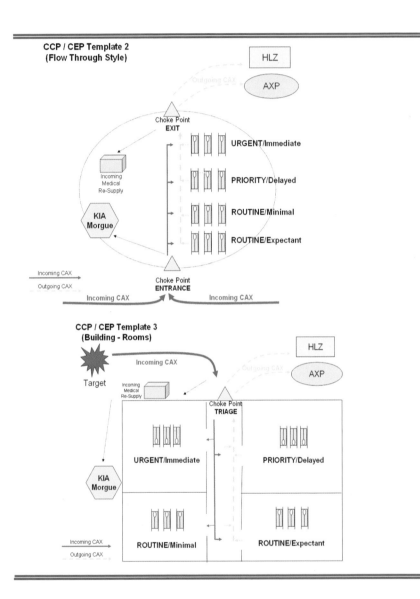

CCP / CEP Template 2
(Flow Through Style)

HLZ

AXP

Choke Point
EXIT

URGENT/Immediate

Incoming
Medical
Re-Supply

PRIORITY/Delayed

KIA
Morgue

ROUTINE/Minimal

ROUTINE/Expectant

Incoming CAX

Outgoing CAX

Choke Point
ENTRANCE

Incoming CAX

Incoming CAX

CCP / CEP Template 3
(Building - Rooms)

HLZ

Incoming CAX

Outgoing CAX

AXP

Target

Incoming
Medical
Re-Supply

Choke Point
TRIAGE

URGENT/Immediate

PRIORITY/Delayed

KIA
Morgue

Incoming CAX

Outgoing CAX

ROUTINE/Minimal

ROUTINE/Expectant

4-12

**CCP / CEP Template 4
(Building – Open/Hanger)**

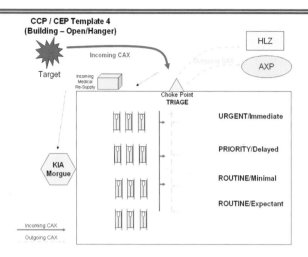

**CCP / CEP Template 5
(Open Area / Field)**

12

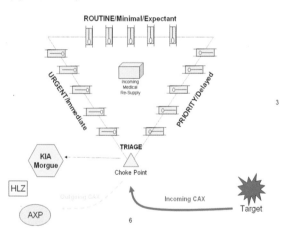

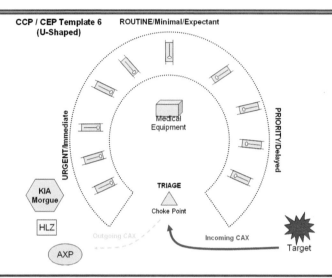

CCP / CEP Template 6
(U-Shaped)

ROUTINE/Minimal/Expectant

URGENT/Immediate

PRIORITY/Delayed

Medical
Equipment

TRIAGE

Choke Point

KIA
Morgue

HLZ

AXP

Outgoing CAX

Incoming CAX

Target

PART 8: General Guidelines for CCP Personnel

- ➢ Maintain Security
- ➢ Maintain Command & Control
- ➢ Maintain Adequate Treatment
- ➢ Maintain Situational Awareness
- ➢ Maintain Organization
- ➢ Maintain Control of Equipment & Supplies
- ➢ Maintain Accountability

PART 9: Casualty Marking and Tagging

- ➢ **COLOR CODING FOR TRIAGE & EVACUATION**
  - Chemlights, colored engineer tape, or triage tags, will be used to color code as follows:

RED	Immediate / Critical (Urgent & Urgent-Surgical)
GREEN	Delayed / Priority
BLUE	Expectant / Routine
NONE	Minimal / Convenience

- ➢ **CASUALTY TAGGING**
  - The casualty card on the following page is the USSOCOM JTF Standard for casualty tagging:

Cax Name_____

Medic's Name_____

Incident: Day or Night

DIRTY	

TIME				
AVPU				
Pulse				
RESP				
BP				

Immediate	Delayed	Expectant	Minimal
RED	GREEN	BLUE	NO CHEM. LT
Critical(Urgent)	Priority	Routine	
<2 hours	<4 hours	<24 hours	

A: NPA   Cric   King LT   ETtube

B: ODressing   NDecompression   ChestTube

C: Tourniquet Hemostatic Packed PressureDx
         SalLock   EJugular   IV   IO

FLUIDS: NS/ RL   **500   1000   1500**
                   Hextend   500   1000

DRUGS:
   PAIN
   ABX
   CWPP

Mech. of Injury- Treatments

PART 10: MEDEVAC Request Format

Use Lines 1-5 for pre-coordinated CASEVAC Requests using JTF Assets

LINE	ITEM	Brevity Codes	
1	Location / Grid	Grid (HLZ Name for JTF Assets)	
2	Frequency & Call-sign of requesting unit	FM Freq Callsign	
3	Number of Patients by Precedence	A – Urgent B – Urgent Surgical C – Priority D – Routine E - Convenience	A – B – C – D – E –
4	Special Equipment Needed	A – None B – Hoist C – Extraction Equipment D – Ventilator	A – B – C – D –
5	Number of Patients by Type (Litter & Ambulatory)	L – # of Litter Patients A - # of Ambulatory Patients	L – A –
6 (Wartime)	Security at Pick-Up Site (Wartime)	N – No enemy troops in area P – Possibly enemy troops in area E – Enemy troops in area (use caution) X – Enemy troops in area (armed escort required)	
6 (Peacetime)	Number and type of wounded, injured or illness	Description of each	
7	Method of Marking Pick-Up Site	A – Panels B – Pyrotechnic Signal C – Smoke Signal D – None E – Other (Specify)	
8	Patient Nationality and Status	A – US Military B – US Civilian C – Non-US Military D – Non-US Civilian E - EPW	
9 (Wartime)	NBC Contamination (Wartime)	N – Nuclear B – Biological C – Chemical	
9 (Peacetime)	Terrain Description (features in and around the landing site)		

Time of Initial MEDEVAC Request: _____

Time of MEDEVAC Launch: _____

Time of MEDEVAC Complete: _____

PART 11: Hazardous Training Medical Coverage

> **DEFINITION**
> - Planning, coordination, and execution of backside medical coverage for high-risk or hazardous training events conducted by Ranger units

> **TYPICAL EVENTS REQUIRING MEDICAL COVERAGE**
> - Airborne operations
> - Fast-rope operations (FRIES)
> - Road Marches (12 miles and over)
> - Maneuver Live Fires
> - Demolitions/Explosives
> - Other

> **MEDICAL COVERAGE DUTIES & RESPONSIBILITIES**

1. **Senior Coverage Medic**
   - Plan & coordinate medical support requirements & considerations
   - Identify Hospitals and evacuation routes
     - Conduct Hospital Site Survey as required
     - Conduct face-to-face with hospital ER
     - Conduct route recon from target to hospital
   - Establish target medical coverage plan and casualty flow
   - Brief OIC/NCOIC medical support plan
     - Clarify OIC/NCOIC responsibilities and guidance
     - Clarify Medical responsibilities and guidance
   - EXECUTION Duties:
     - Patient Treatment & Monitoring on target and en route
     - Advise OIC/NCOIC as required
     - Update OIC/NCOIC/Higher HQ on condition of evacuated casualties
     - Inform unit medical officer of all casualties

2. **OIC / NCOIC of Event**
   - Overall responsible for administrative coverage (including medical)
   - Request / track external medical support requirements
   - Ensure appropriate type and number of vehicles with assigned drivers are dedicated to medical coverage
   - Ensure appropriate communications equipment is allocated to medical personnel
   - Link medical coverage plan with overall administrative coverage plan
   - EXECUTION duties
     - Collect casualty data and report to higher HQs
     - Request MEDEVAC
     - Identify and establish MEDEVAC HLZ

> DETERMINE COVERAGE REQUIREMENTS

- Determine medical support requirements based on type of training and appropriate SOP/Regulation.
  - o RTC 350-2 Airborne SOP (ASOP)
  - o RTC 350-6 FRIESSOP
  - o RTC 350-1-2 (SOSOP)
  - o Local Installation and Range Control Regulations / Guidelines
  - o Training Area specific requirements
- Coordinate and request appropriate equipment, vehicles, personnel, and support assets

DROP ZONE REQUIREMENTS

Medical Support Requirements \ Total Number Of Jumpers	1 to 60	61 to 120	121 to 240	241 to 360	361 to 480	481 to 600	601 to 720	Airland
Medical Officer	N/A	N/A	N/A	N/A	1	1	1	N/A
Senior Medic	1	1	1	1	1	1	1	1
Aidman	N/A	1	2	2	3	3	4	1
Ambulance w/commo	1	1	2	3	4	4	4	1
Communications	1	2	3	3	5	5	6	2
5% Jump Injuries	3	6	12	18	24	30	36	N/A

> MAPS & ROUTE RECONS

- Request/Purchase/Acquire appropriate maps of training areas, adjacent military installations, and cities
  - o Military Grid Reference System (MGRS)
  - o Civilian Maps (Rand McNally, DeLorme, etc...)
  - o Strip Maps / Site Published Maps
- Conduct map and ground recon of training areas (specifically key entrance & exit points).
- Note map problems/errors
- Identify hospitals/fire/EMS locations

- ➢ **IDENTIFY SPECIAL COVERAGE CONSIDERATIONS**
  - Weather
  - Animals
  - Plants
  - Terrain hazards (high angle or high altitude)
- ➢ **IDENTIFY HOSPITALS**
  - Primary and Alternate evacuation hospital
  - One should be a Level 1 Trauma Center
  - Conduct hospital site survey and face-to-face
  - Determine Hospital Communications:
    - o ER Phone Line
    - o ER Ambulance Line
    - o Patient Admin Phone Line
    - o Security Line Phone Line
  - Determine Routes and Directions to hospitals
  - Where are special injuries evacuated?
    - o Neurosurgical
    - o Burns
    - o Trauma Centers
      - Level 1
        - – Neurosurgeon on staff 24 hours
      - Level 2
        - – Neurosurgeon on call, but not on site 24/7
- ➢ **VEHICLE REQUIREMENTS**
  - **Driver:** A dedicated driver – NOT the medic covering the event. Must be familiar with training area and evacuation routes.
  - **Ambulance:** A covered vehicle capable of carrying at least 1 litter with spine-board attached. The vehicle must provide environmental control and adequate space for medical equipment. Mark vehicle as appropriate (ambulance symbols or lights).
    - o Optimal Vehicles:
      - Van (15PAX only)
      - Large SUV (Expedition, Tahoe, etc…)
      - FLA (M996/M997)
    - o Suboptimal Vehicles
      - Open HMMWV / GMV
      - MEDSOV (tactical operations only – not for admin coverage)
      - Small SUV (Explorer, Durango, Cherokee, etc…)
      - Small Van (7PAX)
- ➢ **EQUIPMENT REQUIREMENTS**
  - Standard Medical Equipment
    - o Spinal Immobilization/Stabilization
    - o Splint Sets (Quick Splints)
    - o O2/Masks/BVM

- o Suction, Electric
- o KED/Oregon Spine Splints
- o Traction Splint
- o Vital Signs Monitor (Propaq, PIC, LifePak)
- o Litters (Raven/Skedco/Talon)
- o Blankets
- o MAST
- o Pain Control
- Special Equipment Considerations
  - o Cold Weather
    - REPS (Rescue Wrap & Patient Heaters)
    - Thermal Angels
  - o Hot Weather
    - Fans (battery operated)
    - Cold Packs
  - o Burns

> **COMMUNICATION REQUIREMENTS**
- Equipment
  - o FM & MX frequency capable radios
  - o Cell Phone
- Radio Nets
  - o Administrative Coverage (DZSO Net)
  - o Exercise Target Control (O/C Net)
  - o Tactical Nets
- En route Communications
  - o Cell phone to notify receiving facilities

> **MEDEVAC REQUEST PROCEDURES**
- Military Installation
  - o MEDEVAC unit and location
  - o Request Procedures
    - Range Control?
    - MEDEVAC Freq?
    - Request format (other than 9-Line)
    - Aircraft / HLZ requirements/considerations
- Civilian Life Flight
  - o Contact Numbers & Procedures
    - Direct Line and Alternate Contacts (State Police)
  - o Special Aircraft Considerations
    - Aircraft Capabilities / Limitations
    - Aircraft / HLZ requirements/considerations
- HLZ Marking Requirements

- ➢ **ADMIN CASUALTY FLOW**
  - Point-of-Injury TO Home Station
  - Casualty Flow on the Target / DZ to CCP or HLZ
    - o Tactical to admin link-up and patient turnover
  - From the target to hospital
  - From hospital to home station

General Rule: All casualties go through tactical medical channels unless life, limb, or eyesight is threatened.

- ➢ **TACTICAL DROP ZONE COVERAGE FOR EXERCISES**
  - All casualties go through tactical evacuation channels unless life, limb or eyesight is threatened.
  - No vehicles enter the drop zone without DZSO permission and tactical commanders notification
  - Minimize white lights
  - Minimize impact on tactical operations remaining off the DZ unless directed otherwise
  - If possible, use tactical vehicles/assets to transport to admin CCP sites

- ➢ **PRE-COVERAGE INSPECTIONS**
  - ALWAYS CHECK YOURSELF AND INSPECT SUBORDINATES
  - Inspect / Inventory Medical equipment
    - o Inventory against Hazardous Coverage Checklist
    - o Function check mechanical devices & Monitors
    - o Check Batteries
    - o Aidbags
  - Check Vehicle(s)
    - o PMCS
    - o Fuel Level
    - o Dispatch
    - o Map/Routes
  - Support Equipment
    - o Communications Equipment
    - o Strobe lights / flashlights / head lamps
    - o Night vision
    - o GPS

- ➢ **REHEARSALS**
  - Drive routes to hospitals
    - o During daytime and nighttime
    - o Determine time from target to hospital
    - o Consider civilian traffic interference
  - Conduct target casualty flow to CCP
  - Conduct CCP rehearsal
  - Conduct COMMEX when all sites established

> **TREATMENT DURING EXERCISES**
  - On target
    - U.S. Standard of Care per unit protocols (there is no excuse)
    - Package casualties for evacuation
  - En route
    - Patient Monitoring and re-evaluation of treatment and interventions
    - Notify receiving hospital
  - Inform unit medical officer of casualties
  - Keep OIC/NCOIC informed of patient status with routine updates

PART 12: Pre-Deployment and RRF-1 Assumption

> **EVENTS PRIOR TO DEPLOYMENT & RRF-1 ASSUMPTION**
  - 100% Equipment Inventory and Layout
    - Stockage and Accountability
    - Identify Critical Shortages
  - SRP
    - Unit Medical Readiness (SRP by exception)
    - Individual SRP Packets for assigned medics
  - N-Hour sequence activities review
  - Alert Rosters
  - Plan & POC's for drawing of non-stocked Class VIII
    - NBC Class VIII

> **INVENTORY & LAYOUT**
  - Inspection by Senior Medics of 100% of inventory (equipment & supplies)
  - Complete Layout
  - Shortages Identified and Rectified
  - Re-inspections as necessary
  - Palletize / Load ISU / JI prep

*It is not a waste of time!!! You are not above inspections or PCIs!!!

RMED Equipment Layout Diagram
(Example)

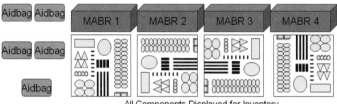

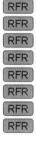

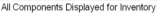

All Components Displayed for Inventory

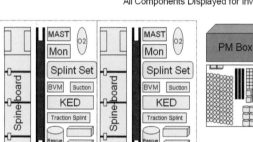

> ## MEDICAL READINESS & SRP
>   - Current Snapshot of Unit in MEDPROS
>   - Identify Med SRP Shortcomings
>   - Advise the Commander on solutions
>   - Plan for the fix
>   - Execute the fix
>   - Update Records
>   - Review / Submit Command Health Report
>   - Review / Submit profile / non-deployable roster
>   - Ensure subordinate medics SRP packets are complete

> ## REVIEW ALERT PROCEDURES
>   - Alert Rosters
>   - N-Hour Sequence review
>   - Who is responsible for what?
>   - Do we have potential short-comings?
>   - Confirm POC's for actions.

> ## MEDICAL LOGISTICS ISSUES
>   - Confirm plan for installation support requirements:
>   - How to draw Class VIII shortages
>   - How to draw NBC Medical Items

- How to conduct a no-notice SRP
- Who do we call for external support?
  - Hospital POCs
  - Installation Support
  - SRP Support
  - Definitive outline of requirements or support needed

PART 13: Post-Deployment and Recovery

- ➤ **AGGRESSIVE LEADERSHIP & MANAGEMENT**
  - The senior medic must take charge and be responsible for his element's post-deployment recovery
  - The senior medic must direct subordinates and enforce standards
  - The senior medic must maintain an air of professionalism
  - Ensure deployment packages are in a high state of readiness

- ➤ **ACCOUNTABILITY OF EQUIPMENT**
  - Hand Receipt items
  - Serial Number items

- ➤ **PMCS / CLEAN / REPAIR EQUIPMENT**
  - Proper Inspection and PMCS on equipment and functions.
  - All equipment cleaned of bodily fluids, environment soiling, and debris.
  - Repair or turn-in broken or malfunctioning equipment.

- ➤ **IDENTIFY & REPLACE SHORTAGES**
  - 100% Inventory of stockages against packing lists
  - Early identification of shortages and expended items
  - Document expenditure trends
  - Submission of request for re-supply
  - Receive supplies
  - Replace stockages
  - 100% Inventory of stockages
  - Maintain shortage list for future stockage

- ➤ **PHASE 1 (Prior to Re-Deployment)**
  - Accountability of sensitive, hand receipt, and serial number items
  - Missing items reported to command immediately.
  - Damaged items reported to command immediately
  - Remove batteries from equipment.
  - Pack sensibly into ISU-90 or onto pallets.

- ➤ **PHASE 2 (Days 1 to 2 of Recovery)**
  - Complete unit individual requirements-weapons, NVG's, P-mask, commo
  - Disseminate Recovery Plan and Schedule
  - Disseminate Post-Deployment SRP Plan

- o Anti-Malarial Prophylaxis
- o Lab Testing required (HIV, etc…)
- o Post-Deployment Health Surveillance Forms
- Conduct Individual Inventories
  - o RMED Aid Bags
  - o Individual Ranger BCKs
  - o Squad RFR Bags
  - o Utilize PSG & SL to get platoon/squad inspections & requirements
- Turn In Narcotics and Prescriptions/FMC's
- Submit individual shortages

- ➢ **PHASE 3 (Days 3 to 4 of Recovery)**
  - Receive and re-stock individual items
    - o RMED aid bags
    - o Ranger BCKs
    - o Squad RFR Bags
    - o Replace/Recharge all batteries
  - Clean/Inspect/PMCS Medical Equipment
    - o Hazardous Coverage Kits
      - • All items cleaned, function checked, and component inventory
    - o Inventory MABR Sets
      - • Remove all items
      - • Clean Pelicans
      - • Re-Pack available components fixing immediate shortages as available
      - • Re-Assess Shortages
    - o Inventory PM and Contingency Boxes (same protocol)
  - Submit Shortages for MABR, Hazardous Coverage Kits, PM & Contingency boxes

- ➢ **PHASE 4 (Days 5 to 7 of Recovery)**
  - Receive requested shortages
  - Restock Individual Items, MABR, Hazardous Coverage Kits, PM & Contingency boxes
  - Reassess shortages and ensure long-term order is initiated.

- ➢ **PHASE 5 (NLT Day 9 of Recovery)**
  - All Post-Deployment SRP Requirements completed.
    - o Post-Deployment Health Surveillance Surveys turned into higher.
    - o All labs and prophylaxis requirements completed or scheduled
  - Inspection from Next-Higher Med Supervisor
    - o 100% layout, inventory, and inspection of medical equipment and supplies
    - o Re-sign/Re-assess hand receipts. Initiate report of surveys as required.
    - o Post-Inspection Corrections initiated
- Schedule AAR and Counseling periods

> **PHASE 6 (NLT Day 15 of Recovery)**
- Conduct AAR/Lessons Learned
  - All medical personnel in unit
  - Every man comes to the table with:
    - 3 X Sustains
    - 3 X Improves
    - 1 X Lesson Learned
  - Document AAR Findings, archive findings, and submit to higher.
- Counseling
  - Focus on performance during the period of the deployment.
  - Offer guidance & recommendations
  - Provide every individual with at least:
    - 2 X Areas to Sustain
    - 2 X Areas to Improve
    - 1 X Learning Assignment

SECTION FIVE

RMED
PACKING LISTS
&
REFERENCE

The packing lists below are intended to be minimum stockage lists for the typical Ranger combat mission. Medics are authorized the flexibility to ADD components to their equipment as based on the mission requirements. Medics are not authorized to deviate from the minimum packing list unless approved by the unit medical director. Individual line item deviations are authorized for items that are unavailable through Class VIII channels as long as replacement items are merely a deviation from a specific brand name or manufacturer.

RMED RBA / RLCS Minimum Stockage

The RMED RBA/RLCS packing list are items that the medic carries on his body without opening an aid-bag or rucksack. All items are to be carried in a manner that provides ease of access. The intent of this packing list is to provide all immediate initial care for a trauma casualty without opening external bags and equipment.

NSN	COMMON NAME	QTY
	RMED Kit, Ranger Load Carriage System (RLCS)	1
AIRWAY		
6515-01-540-7568	Cricothyroidotomy Kit	1
6515-01-529-1187	Nasopharyngeal Airway, 28fr w/Lubricant	1
BREATHING		
6515-01-541-0635	14G / 3.5" Needle	1
6515-01-532-8019	Chest Seal (Hyfin) 6"	2
6510-01-408-1920	Chest Seal (Asherman)	2
CIRCULATION / BLEEDING		
6515-01-521-7976	Combat Applications Tourniquet (CAT)	2
6510-01-492-2275	Emergency Trauma Dressing, 6"	2
6510-01-541-2896	Hemostatic Dressing (Chitosan)	2
6510-01-541-2896	Hemostatic Bandage (Chitoflex)	1
6510-01-529-1213	Kerlex, Vacuum Sealed	4
DISABILITY / IMMOBILIZATION		
		0
FLUIDS / IV ACCESS		
6515-01-537-4094	Saline Lock Kit	2
Local Purchase	Sharps Container	1
MONITORING & DIAGNOSTIC		
Local Purchase	Pulsoximeter, Finger	1
MISCELLANEOUS		
6515-01-540-7284	Exam Light (Tactical Green)	1
Local Purchase	Headlamp	1
NSN by size	Gloves, Exam (Black Talon)	6
6515-01-538-9276	Trauma Shears, 7.25"	1
6515-01-540-7226	Scissor Leash or Gear-Keeper	1

RMED Assault Aid-Bag Minimum Stockage

NSN	COMMON NAME	QTY
6545-01-539-6444	AidBag, M-9 (TSS-M-9-RG)	1
AIRWAY		
6515-01-529-1187	Nasopharyngeal Airway, 28fr w/Lubricant	1
6515-01-540-7568	Cricothyroidotomy Kit	1
6515-01-515-0151	King LT-D Supralayrngeal Airway size 4	1
6515-01-540-7206	Suction, Hand-held (Suction Easy or Squid)	1
BREATHING		
6515-01-541-0635	14G / 3.5" Needle	1
6515-01-532-8019	Chest Seal (Hyfin) 6"	2
6510-01-408-1920	Chest Seal (Asherman)	2
6515-01-519-4476	Bag-Valve-Mask	1
CIRCULATION / BLEEDING		
6515-01-521-7976	Combat Applications Tourniquet (CAT)	2
6510-01-492-2275	Emergency Trauma Dressing, 6"	3
6510-01-541-8121	Emergency Trauma Dressing, Abdominal	1
6510-01-502-6938	Hemostatic Dressing (Chitosan)	2
6510-01-541-2896	Hemostatic Bandage (Chitoflex)	2
6510-01-529-1213	Kerlex, Vacuum Sealed	3
Pending	Tactical Compression Wrap	1
DISABILITY / IMMOBILIZATION		
6510-00-201-1755	Cravat Bandage, Muslin (or ACE Wrap)	2
6515-01-346-9186	Traction Splint (KTD or TTS)	1
6515-01-494-1951	SAM Splint II	2
FLUIDS / IV ACCESS		
6515-01-537-4094	Saline Lock Kit	2
6505-01-498-8636	Hextend IV 500cc	2
NSN	Sodium Choride Flush, 50cc	1
Component List	IV Kit	3
6515-01-530-6147	FAST-1 Sternal Intraosseous	1
6515-01-537-2611	BOA Constricting Band	1
6515-01-523-3317	Raptor IV Securing Device	3
Local Purchase	Sharps Shuttle Container w/Locking Mechanism	1
MONITORING & DIAGNOSTIC		
Local Purchase	Stethoscope (mission dependent)	1
Local Purchase	Pulsoximeter, Finger	1
MEDICATIONS		
Component List	RMED Medications Kit	1
EVACUATION EQUIPMENT		
6515-01-532-8056	Hypothermia Kit (mission and aidbag dependent)	1
MISCELLANEOUS		
6515-01-540-7284	Exam Light (Tactical Green)	1
NSN for size	Gloves, Exam (Black Talon)	6
6510-01-532-4283	Tape, 2"	2
6515-01-538-9276	Trauma Shears, 7.25"	1
6515-01-540-7226	Scissor Leash or Gear-Keeper	1

	MISSION DEPENDENT AIDBAG ITEMS	
Component List	Chest Tube Kit (Mission Dependent)	1
6515-01-509-6866	SAM Pelvic Sling	1
6515-01-541-8147	ACE Cervical Collar	1
6515-01-148-6178	Field Otoscope/Opthalmoscope Set	1
Component List	Minor Wound Care Kit	1
Local Purchase	Glucometer	1
6515-00-149-1406	Thermometer, Oral	1
6515-00-149-1407	Thermometer, Rectal	1
		0
		0

RMED Medications Kit Minimum Stockage

RMED MEDICATIONS KIT (Proficient and Always Carried)		
Local Purchase	Drug Case (Otter or Armadillo)	1
Component List	Combat Wound Pill Pack (CWPP)	2
6505-01-091-7538	Diphenhydramine HCL Inj 50mg (Benadryl)	1
6505-01-492-6420	Dexamethasone Inj, 4mg/ml (5ml) (Decadron)	1
6505-01-238-5634	Epi-Pen Anaphylaxis Auto-Injector	1
NDC 63459-0508-30	Fentanyl Transmuccosal Lozenge, 800mcg	4
6505-01-503-5374	Ertapenem Inj, 1gm (Invanz)	2
6505-00-149-0113	Morphine Sulfate Inj, 5mg	5
6505-01-435-9958	Nalaxone Inj, 0.4mg (Narcan)	5
6505-00-680-7352	Promethazine Inj, 25mg (Phenergan)	5
NDC 0074-3795-01	Ketorolac Inj, 30mg (Toradol)	2
6505-01-199-3137	Acetaminophen Tabs, 500mg (Tylenol)	25
6505-00-137-5891	Diazepam Inj, 5mg (Valium)	2
6515-01-344-8487	Tubex Injector, Cartridge Unit	1
6515-01-356-8511	Syringe, 10cc Luer-Lok Tip	5
NSN	Needle, Hypo 18G/1.5"	5

COMBAT WOUND PILL PACK (CWPP) Carried by every Ranger		
6505-01-199-3137	Acetaminophen Tabs, 500mg (Tylenol)	2
NDC 0085-1733-01	Moxifloxacin HCL Tab, 400mg (Avelox)	1
6505-01-541-3243	Meloxicam, 15mg Tab (Mobic)	1

SALINE LOCK KIT (6515-01-537-4094)

NSN	18G X 1.5" Catheter/Needle	2
6510-00-786-3736	Alcohol Pad	2
6515-01-519-6764	Constricting Band, Penrose	1
6510-00-058-4421	2X2 Sponge, Sterile	1
6515-01-321-3336	Saline Plug, Locking	1
6515-01-356-8511	Syringe, 10cc Luer-Lok Tip	1
NSN	18G X 1.5" Needle, Hypodermic	1
6515-01-523-3317	Raptor IV Securing Band	1
6510-01-135-4267	Tega-derm	1
8105-01-099-0355	Pill Bag	1

CHEST TUBE KIT

6515-00-334-9500	Forceps, 9" Pean	1
6515-01-149-8097	Scalpel, #10	1
6515-00-763-7366	36fr Chest Tube	1
6515-00-926-9150	Heimlich Valve	1
6510-00-721-9808	Sponge, Sterile 4X4	4
6510-01-408-1920	Asherman Chest Seal	0
NSN	Chux	1
6505-00-598-6116	Lidocaine Inj, 1%	1
6515-01-356-8511	Syringe, 10cc Luer-Lok Tip	1
6510-01-532-4283	Tape, 2"	1
NSN	Sterile Gloves	2
NSN	1-O Armed Suture	2
6510-00-202-0800	Petrolatum Gauze	2
6505-00-914-3593	Betadine Solution .5 oz	0

CRICOTHYROIDOTOMY KIT (6515-01-540-7568)

6515-01-149-8097	Scalpel, #10	1
NSN by size	Gloves, Exam (Black Talon)	2
6515-01-356-8511	Syringe, 10cc Luer-Lok Tip	1
Pending	Tracheal Hook (NARP)	1
6510-00-786-3736	Alcohol Prep Pad	1
6510-01-010-0307	Povidine-Iodine Pad	1
Pending	Tube, 6mm Bore-cuffed Cricothyroidotomy	1

IV KIT

6515-00-115-0032	IV Solution Set, 10 drops/ml	1
6515-01-537-4094	Saline Lock Kit	1
6510-01-135-4267	Tegaderm 4.75"X4"	1

MINOR WOUND CARE KIT		
6510-00-111-0708	Pad, Non-Adherent (Telfa)	4
6505-00-914-3593	Betadine 0.5oz	2
6510-01-456-2000	Moleskin, 12"	1
6510-00-597-7469	Band-Aids 3"X.75"	10
6510-00-054-7255	Steri-Strips	5
6510-00-721-9808	Sponge, 4X4 Sterile	5
6515-01-149-8097	Scalpel, #10	2
6510-01-010-0307	Pad, Povidine	5
6510-00-786-3736	Pad, Alcohol	5
Local Purchase	Compeed Dressing	5
6505-01-414-1821	Tincture of Benzoin Ampule 0.6ml	5
6510-01-008-7917	Applicator, Povidine-Iodine	2

ABBREVIATION LIST

AAS	acute abdominal series	C/O	complaining of
ABD	abdomen	CLS	combat lifesaver
ABG	arterial blood gas	CMD	command
AC	before eating (ante cibium)	CMO	civil-military operations
ACL	anterior cruciate ligament	CNS	central nervous system
ACLS	Advanced Cardiac Life Support	CO	commanding officer
A&O X -	alert and oriented times orientation	CO	carbon monoxide
AF	afebrile	CO2	carbon dioxide
AFSOC	US Air Force Special Operations Command	COTCCC	committee on tactical combat casualty care
AKA	above-the-knee amputation	CPAP	continuous positive airway pressure
ALS	advanced life support	CPR	cardiopulmonary resuscitation
AP	anteroposterior	CR	casualty response
AMEDD	army medical department	CRTRL	casualty response training for ranger leaders
AMS	acute mountain sickness; altered mental status	CSF	cerebral spinal fluid
		CTA	clear to auscultation
ARDS	acute respiratory distress syndrome	CXP	casualty exchange point
		CXR	chest x-ray
ASA	acetylsalicylic acid (aspirin)	D/C	discontinue or discharge
ASAP	as soon as possible	DDx	differential diagnosis
AT/NC	atraumatic, normocephalic	DEA	drug enforcement agency
ATLS	advanced trauma life support	DMO	diving medical officer
ATM	advanced trauma manager	DOA	dead on arrival
ATP	advanced tactical practitioner	DOB	date of birth
AXP	ambulance exchange point	DOE	dyspnea on exertion
BAS	battalion aid station	DNBI	disease/non-battle injury
bid	twice a day	DNR	do not resuscitate
BCK	bleeder control kit	DO	doctor of osteopathy
BKA	below-the-knee amputation	DOB	date of birth
BLS	basic life support	DPL	diagnostic peritoneal lavage
BM	bowel movement	DPN	drops per minute
BN	battalion	DPT	diphtheria, pertussis, tetanus
BP	blood pressure	DTR	deep tendon reflex
BPM	beats per minute	DVT	deep venous thrombosis
BRBPR	bright red blood per rectum	Dx	diagnosis
BS	bowel sounds	DZ	drop zone
BSI	body substance isolation	EBL	estimated blood loss
BVM	bag-valve-mask	ECG	electrocardiogram
BW	biological warfare	EDC	estimated date of confinement
Bx	biopsy	EKG	electrocardiogram
c	with (cum)	EMG	electromyelogram
C	celsius or centigrade	EMS	emergency medical system or service
C2	command & control	EMT	emergency medical technician
CA	civil affairs	EMT-B	emergency medical technician-basic
CAD	coronary artery disease	EMT-I	emergency medical technician-intermediate
CAM	chemical agent monitor	EMT-P	emergency medical technician-paramedic
CAMS	civil affairs medical sergeant	EOM	extraocular muscles
CANA	convulsant antidote for nerve agents	EOMI	extraocular muscles intact
CAT	computed axial tomography	EPW	enemy prisoner of war
CAT	combat application tourniquet	ET	endotracheal (tube)
CAX	casualties	ETOH	ethanol alcohol
CBC	complete blood count	F	farenheit
cc	cubic centimeter	FB	foreign body
CC	chief complaint	F&D	fixed and dilated
CCP	casualty collection point	FamHx	family history
CDC	centers for disease control	F/C	fevers, chills
CDR	commander	FDA	food and drug administration
CEP	casualty evacuation point	FITT	frequency, intensity, time, type
CHI	closed head injury	FMED	flight medic

FP	family practice	LASER	light amplification by stimulated emission of
FRAGO	fragmentation order		radiation
F/U	follow-up	LBP	low back pain
FUO	fever of unknown origin	LE	lower extremities
Fx	fracture	LIH	left inguinal hernia
G	gram(s)	LLL	left lower lobe
G	guage (needle)	LMP	last menstrual period
GCS	glascow coma scale	LOC	loss of consciousness
GERD	gastroesophageal reflux disease	LOD	line of duty
GI	gastrointestinal	LP	lumbar puncture
GPS	global positioning system	LR	lactated ringers
GSW	gunshot wound	LLQ	left lower quadrant
gtt	drops	LUL	left upper lobe
GU	genitourinary	LUQ	left upper quadrant
HA	headache	MAPCODE	Monitor, Antibiotics, Pain Control, Contact MO,
HACE	high altitude cerebral edema		Oxygen, Document, Evacuate
HAHO	high altitude, high opening	MAST	military anti-shock trousers
	(parachute)	MC	medical control
HALO	high altitude, low opening	MC	medical corps
	(parachute)	MI	myocardial infarction
HAPE	high altitude pulmonary edema	MOI	mechanism of injury
Hct	hematocrit	mmHg	millimeters of mercury
HE	high explosive	MMR	measles, mumps, rubella
HEENT	head, eyes, ears, nose, throat	MO	medical officer
Hg	mercury	MOUT	military operations in urban terrain
Hgb	hemoglobin	MRI	magnetic resonance imaging
HLZ	helicopter landing zone	MVA	motor vehicle accident
HPI	history of present illness	NAD	no acute distress
Hr	hour	NAEMT	national association of emergency medical
HR	heart rate		technicians
HS	bed time (hours of sleep)	NEO	non-combatant evacuation operation
HSV	herpes simplex virus	NKA	no known allergies
HTN	hypertension	NKDA	no known drug allergies
HTS	hypertonic saline	NPA	nasopharyngeal airway
Hx	history	NPO	nothing by mouth (nil per os)
IAPP	inspection, auscultation, palpation,	NS	normal saline
	percussion	NREMT	national registry of emergency medical
IAW	in accordance with…		technicians
ICW	in conjunction with…	NSAID	nonsteroidal antiinflammatory drug
I&D	incision and drainage	NSR	normal sinus rhythm
ID	infectious disease	NTG	nitroglycerin
IDC	independent duty corpsman (USN)	N/V/D	nausea, vomiting, diarrhea
IDMT	independent duty medical technician	OB	obstetrics
	(USAF)	OCOKA	observation and fire, concealment and cover,
IM	intramuscular		obstacles, key terrain, and avenues of
I&O	intake and output		approach
IPPB	intermittent positive pressure	OD	right eye (oculus dexter), overdose
	breathing	OE	otitis externa
IV	intravenous	OM	otitis media
JOMAC	judgement, orientation, mentation,	OPA	oralpharyngeal airway
	abstraction, calculation	OPORD	operations order
JVD	jugular venous distention	OPQRST	onset, provokes, quality, radiates, severity, time
JCCP	joint casualty collection point	OPV	oral polio vaccine
JSOC	joint special operations command	OS	left eye (oculus sinister)
JSOMTC	joint special operations medical	OTSG	office of the surgeon general
	training center	PA	physician assistant
kg	kilogram	PAX	personnel
K	potassium	PC	precious cargo (operational)
KIA	killed in action	PC	after eating (post cibum)
L	left	PCN	penicillin
LA	lymphadenopathy	PE	physical exam or pulmonary embolism
lac	laceration	PEA	pulseless electrical activity

PERRLA	pupils equal, round, reactive to light and accomadation	Rx	prescription, treatment
PFT	pulmonary function test	s	without (sine)
PHTLS	pre-hospital trauma life support	S1	personnel and administration
PJ	USAF pararescuemen	S2	intelligence and security
PM	preventive medicine	S3	operations and training
PMHx	past medical history	S4	logistics and supply
PMI	point of maximal impulse	S5	civil affairs and information operations
PO	by mouth (per os)	S6	signal and communications
POW	prisoner of war	S8	force modernization, plan, R&D
PPD	purified protein derivative	SCUBA	self-contained underwater breathing apparatus
ppm	parts per million	SEM	systolic ejection murmur
PPV	positive pressure ventilation	SF	special forces
PR	per rectum	SFMS	special forces medical sergeant
PRN	as often as needed (pro re nata)	SL	sublingual
PSHx	past surgical history	SRMED	senior ranger medic
PSI	pounds per square inch	Sn	signs
Pt	patient	SocHx	social history
PT	physical therapist	SOAR	special operations aviation regiment
PUD	peptic ulcer disease	SOB	shortness of breath
PULHES	physical profile factors: P-physical capacity or stamina, U-upper extremities, L-lower extremities, H-hearing and ears, E-eyes, S-psychiatric	SOCM	special operations combat medic
		SOF	special operations forces
		SQ	subcutaneous
		STD	sexually transmitted disease
		Surg	Surgeon (Battalion, Regimental, or command)
q	every (quaque)	Sx	symptoms
QC	quality control	Tab	tablet
qd	every day	TBD	to be determined
qh	every hour	TBSA	total body surface area
q _h	every _ hours	TCCC	tactical combat casualty care
qid	four times a day (quater in die)	TC3	tactical combat casualty care
qod	every other day	Td	tetanus-diphtheria toxoid
qt	quart	tid	three times a day (ter in die)
qty	quantity	TKO	to keep open
R	right	TM	tympanic membrane
RBC	red blood cell	TMT	trauma management team
RDA	recommended dietary allowance	TNTC	to numerous to count
REM	rapid eye movement	tsp	teaspoon
RFR	ranger first responder	TTP	tenderness to palpation
Rh	Rhesus blood factor	Tx	treatment
RHQ	regimental headquarters	ud	as directed (ut dictum)
RGR	ranger	UE	upper extremities
RIH	right inguinal hernia	URI	upper respiratory tract infection
RLL	right lower lobe	USASOC	united states army special operations command
RLQ	right lower quadrant	USSOCOM	united states special operations command
RMED	ranger medic	UTI	urinary tract infection
RMED	regimental medical section	VA	visual acuity
RML	right middle lobe	VD	venereal disease
R/O	rule out	VSS	vital signs stable
ROM	range of motion	WARNORD	warning order
ROS	review of systems	WBC	white blood cell
RSTB	regimental special troops battalion	WHO	world health organization
RUL	right upper lobe	WD	well developed
RUQ	right upper quadrant	WIA	wounded in action
RR	respiratory rate	WMD	weapons of mass destruction
RRF-1	ranger ready force one	WN	well nourished
RRF-2	ranger ready force two	WNL	within normal limits
RRF-3	ranger ready force three	WP	white phosphorus
RRR	regular rate and rhythm	XO	executive officer
RSRMED	regimental senior medic	Y/O	years old
RSURG	regimental surgeon	1SG	first sergeant
RTC	return to clinic	91W	army military occupational specialty - health care specialist

| 68W | army military occupational specialty - health care specialist as of 01 Oct 06 |
| >,<,= | greater than, less than, equal |

Conversion Charts

Length Conversions

1 inch = 2.54 cm

1 foot = 30.5 cm = 0.305 m

1 yard = 0.91 m

1 mile = 1.6 km

1 mm = 0.1 cm = 0.039 in

1 cm = 10 mm = 0.39 in

1 m = 100 cm = 39 in

1 km = 100 m = 1093 yd

Weight Conversions

1 oz = 30 g

1 lb = 16 oz = 0.45 kg

1 ton = 2000 lbs = 907 kg

1 grain = 65 mg

1 g = 001 kg = 0.36 oz

1 kg = 1000 g = 2.2 lbs

1 ton (metric) = 1000 kg = 2200 lbs

Body Weight Conversions (Pounds to Kilogram)

110 lb	49.89 kg
120 lb	54.43 kg
130 lb	58.96 kg
140 lb	63.50 kg
150 lb	68.04 kg
160 lb	72.57 kg
170 lb	77.11 kg
180 lb	81.64 kg
190 lb	86.18 kg
200 lb	90.72 kg

Volume Conversions

1 fl oz = 30 ml = 30 cc

1 US Gal = 128 fl oz = 3785 ml

1 cc = 0.001 liter

1 ml = 1 cc = 0.34 fl oz

1 liter = 1000 ml = 340 fl oz

Temperature Conversions

F = (1.8) X C + 32

C = (F – 32) / (1.8)

The Ranger Medic Code

1. I will always remember that these are the finest Infantry on this earth, and that as such they deserve the finest health care.

2. No Ranger or Ranger dependent who comes to me for health care will ever be turned away without their needs being addressed, even if their paperwork/administrative requirements are not in order.

3. I will never let slip my mind the fact that in chaos of battle, I am all that stands between that bleeding, wounded Ranger and the finality of death. I will perform my job with such skill that the grim reaper will walk away empty-handed.

4. I will always remember that I must not only treat wounded Rangers, I must also carry them sometimes. I will maintain the physical conditioning necessary to accomplish this.

5. I will always remember that uniforms, weapons and supplies can all be DX'd but that each Ranger only comes with one body. I will never jeopardize the safety and/or recovery of that body by performing medical tasks beyond my skill and training.

6. I will always be cognizant of the fact that people do not suddenly get well after 1700 hours and on weekends, and that as such, I will willingly provide or coordinate for health care 24 hours a day, 7 days a week.

7. I will never do anything stupid because "they" or "regulations" require it to be so. I will find a way to accomplish my mission and serve the Rangers of this Regiment.

8. I will always remember that everything I use is paid for by US citizens. I will remember those tax dollars are collected from the American people and given to the Rangers because those people believe that in exchange for that money they will be kept safe from the tyrants of the world.

9. I will never forget that this is an Infantry unit supported by a medical team; not a medical team supported by a plethora of Infantry.

10. I will never forget that when the tyrants of the earth look towards the USA and plot mischief, they see a wall of cold steel backed up by determined men wearing Tan Berets; and then they plot their mischief somewhere else. The extent to which I support that wall is the extent to which I have a right to consume oxygen.

"It is not the strongest of the species that survive, but the one most responsive to change"
-Charles Darwin

"Greater love has no one than this, that he lay down his life for his friends."
-John 15:13 (NIV)

"The quality of a person's life is in direct proportion to their commitment to excellence, regardless of their chosen endeavor"
-Vince Lombardi

"To know what you know and to know what you don't know, that is knowledge"
-Confucius

The Ranger Creed

Recognizing that I volunteered as Ranger, fully knowing the hazards of my chosen profession, I will always endeavor to uphold the prestige, honor, and high esprit de corps of my Ranger Regiment.

Acknowledging the fact that a Ranger is a more elite soldier who arrives at the cutting edge of battle by land, sea, or air, I accept the fact that as a Ranger, my country expects me to move further, faster and fight harder than any other soldier.

Never shall I fail my comrades. I will always keep myself mentally alert, physically strong, and morally straight and I will shoulder more than my share of the task whatever it may be, one hundred percent and then some.

Gallantly will I show the world that I am a specially selected and well trained soldier. My courtesy to superior officers, neatness of dress, and care of equipment shall set the example for others to follow.

Energetically will I meet the enemies of my country. I shall defeat them on the field of battle for I am better trained and will fight with all my might. Surrender is not a Ranger word. I will never leave a fallen comrade to fall into the hands of the enemy, and under no circumstances will I ever embarrass my country.

Readily will I display the intestinal fortitude required to fight on to the Ranger objective and complete the mission, though I be the lone survivor.

Rangers Lead the Way